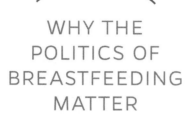

WHY THE POLITICS OF BREASTFEEDING MATTER

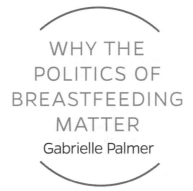

WHY THE POLITICS OF BREASTFEEDING MATTER

Gabrielle Palmer

pinter & martin

Why the Politics of Breastfeeding Matter (Pinter & Martin Why It Matters: 7)

First published by Pinter & Martin Ltd 2016

© 2016 Gabrielle Palmer

With additional material by Yasmin Hosny

ISBN 978-1-78066-525-2
Also available as ebook

Pinter & Martin Why It Matters ISSN 2056-8657

Series editor: Susan Last
Index: Helen Bilton

British Library Cataloguing-in-Publication Data
A catalogue record for this book is available from the British Library.

Set in Minion

Printed and bound in the UK by Ashford Colour Press Ltd, Gosport, Hampshire

This book has been printed on paper that is sourced and harvested from sustainable forests and is FSC accredited.

Pinter & Martin Ltd
6 Effra Parade
London SW2 1PS

pinterandmartin.com

Contents

This book is dedicated to the memory
of Dr Zef Ebrahim (1932–2013)
who spoke truth to power

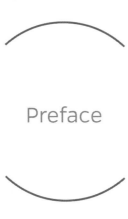

Preface

In 1974 I read a booklet called *The Baby Killer*.[1] Its contents shocked me. I learned that a woman with young children, just like me, could be tricked into buying a product that caused the death of her baby. This was such a clearcut issue I assumed it could be sorted in five years... I was young. I got involved. Twelve years later childbirth educator Sheila Kitzinger asked me to write a book called *The Politics of Breastfeeding*.[2] It's now in its third edition and, tragically, still relevant. I still believe that of all the problems that beset our world this one could be easily resolved. If you want to know more read the bigger book. This is just a tiny taster of why the politics of breastfeeding matter; I hope it will inspire you to find out more and to take action.

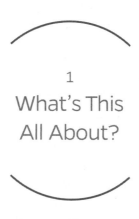

1
What's This
All About?

There is only one reason that a woman should not breastfeed, and that is if she doesn't want to.

Sheila Kitzinger (1929–2015)

At her New Year party, my friend introduced me to her aunt, Fiona,[*] a highly educated, posh woman: 'This is Gabrielle, she's a world expert on breastfeeding'. 'How ghastly!' said Fiona, with feeling. Afterwards my friend and I laughed. I was used to this. Generally when asked what I do, I mumble something about nutrition. I get too worn out by the emotion, both negative and positive, this topic provokes. In this book I'm going to tell you why it is a 'ghastly subject' indeed but not quite in the way Fiona meant.

---

[*] All names have been changed.

How to get rich and famous

If you invented a product that was both a delicious and nutritious food, and a wonder drug that protected the consumers from illness, making them grow healthier and more beautiful every day, you would become rich and famous. If you could manufacture this product out of cheap, everyday materials and could deliver it on request at a moment's notice, you would become a multi-billionaire. Moreover, if every mouthful could adapt to each consumer's changing needs and have health benefits that last a lifetime, you might win a big award, a Nobel Prize perhaps, for your scientific and economic genius. You would have created the world's first personalised medicine for the most important time of life. Something science is striving to achieve.

At least half of you can already do this,* and many of you are or once did. But I lied about the money and the prizes. Women have been breastfeeding since the dawn of human existence, but are the poorest and least powerful half of humanity.

The people who get extremely rich, the companies who make and sell artificial milks, produce an inferior product and delivery system, but have convinced us it is as good or better than the original.

'But, but,' I hear you shout, 'what about all the women who can't breastfeed. Don't their babies starve to death? Lots of women can't feed** and lots of babies cannot be

---

* I hope half of you are male readers.
** Women avoid breastfeeding, or stop early, for many reasons discussed throughout this book. Limiting time at the breast and poor attachment are the main causes of pain and lactation going

breastfed. What about women in famines? Or those who are ill, have died, or are just not around? What about orphans and adoptions? Anyway, my mum couldn't feed me, her nipples were the wrong shape. What if there are quadruplets? What about work? Mothers can't go out to work and breastfeed! You're not telling me that women should stay at home? Besides, it's awful. I tried to feed, but it was agony and anyway my baby never settled. The best thing I ever did was put him on the bottle.'

Let's all take a deep breath right now. Yes, many women have had bad experiences, but it doesn't have to be like this. Let's ask ourselves why almost all Scandinavian women breastfeed and only around half of Irish women even start? Why do so many women in rich countries 'try' and give up within a few days or weeks when women in some of the poorest societies cannot believe that a woman could 'fail' to breastfeed? Let's ask ourselves why it is one of the few positive health behaviours more common in poor countries than in rich ones? And let's ask ourselves why, if breastfeeding is the 'gold standard' for a child, has replacing it with sub-standard products become so normal?

Does it matter?

Yes it does. Breastfeeding is vital for the health and wellbeing of our global society in so many ways. Whether a child is breastfed or not is a question of sickness and

---

wrong. Cultural and medical ignorance lead to a lack of skilled support, perpetuated myths and destruction of confidence. For example, women with flat nipples were told they could not breastfeed. Untrue. The entrenched culture of artificial feeding has been shaped by relentless marketing.

health in the rich world* and a matter of life and death in the poorest regions. Breastfeeding can be an important equaliser within and across societies.

Does it make a difference?

Yes it does. The outcomes of breastfeeding** are universal, but the consequences of *not* breastfeeding differ depending on where in the world a child is born. Children born into poverty suffer the risks of malnutrition, sickness and early death significantly more than those born with access to wealth and healthcare. The longer-term consequences of not being breastfed, such as malnutrition, poorer growth and development, obesity, diabetes and much more, hurt the poorest the most. And this is just at the individual level. Multiply this effect across populations, and we see how the positive difference breastfeeding makes is becoming more and more important in a world besieged by humanitarian and environmental crises. Three major issues of our time are mass migration, antibiotic resistance and climate change. Breastfeeding impacts them all but I'll leave these topics until the end.

Everyday killers

The commonest killers of babies worldwide are pneumonia (respiratory infection or RI) and diarrhoea

---

* If you earn more than $28,000 (£18,200) per year, you are in the richest 5% of the world's population. Someone earning just $11,000 (£7,000) per year is living below the US poverty line, but is still richer than 85% of people in the world.[3]

** This book is too short to include all the evidence about the outcomes of breastfeeding and risks of not breastfeeding, but see Appendix 1 for a summary.

> *A millionaire's baby who is not breastfed is less healthy than an exclusively breastfed baby whose mother is in the poorest social group.*
> J Stewart Forsyth, Ninewells Medical School, Scotland 2006

(gastro-intestinal infection or GI). The less breastfeeding and the more artificial feeding a baby gets, the greater her risk of getting one of these infections. Until the 1990s many scientists and doctors claimed that feeding method made no difference to health in rich countries. Then researchers uncovered, to their astonishment, the evidence that infection rates (GI and RI) for artificially fed babies in clean, cool Dundee in Scotland were equal to those of artificially fed babies in the hot, crowded slums of Manila in the Philippines. Because of rapid diagnosis and treatment in an excellent health system, the Dundee babies quickly recovered and survived, but in Manila, where services were overstretched, sickness was more severe and death rates high.

Despite a welcome fall in child deaths, six million under-fives still die each year worldwide. Of these 823,000 are lost either because they're not breastfed at all, or because breastfeeding is delayed or restricted, or stopped too early.[4] That's more than 2,000 baby deaths each day that could be prevented through optimal breastfeeding practices. 'Optimal' means exclusive breastfeeding (no water, juices, milks or sloppy foods) in the first six months and then continued breastfeeding, together with nutritious family foods, for two years or beyond. Such optimal breastfeeding practices would also benefit women's health, preventing an extra 20,000 annual deaths from breast cancer globally.

All this sickness and death is not because mothers cannot produce breastmilk. The proportion of women who really cannot produce milk is so tiny that few of my colleagues have met one case in a lifetime.* It is because artificial milks and other substitutes for breastfeeding do not just replace the ideal food with an inferior one, but can actually introduce infection and deprive the baby of his full quota of infection fighting factors.** Much illness and death could be prevented if families and health professionals realised that the less a baby is breastfed and the more she is artificially fed, the higher her risk of infection.***

Globally, if all babies were breastfed within an hour of birth, 22 per cent of newborn deaths would be prevented.[5] An infant breastfed within an hour of birth is three times more likely to survive than one breastfed

---

* Sheehan's syndrome, when the mother's pituitary gland has been damaged, is one rare cause. If a woman has no milk after birth it is a sign of a fragment of retained placenta, a life-threatening condition requiring rapid treatment.

** This protection is amazing. Breastmilk already contains antibodies against all the diseases a mother has met in her own lifetime, but her body is continually manufacturing new antibodies that go into her milk when she and her baby meet new infections.

*** Breastmilk also contains general protection. For example, a protein called immunoglobulin A (IgA) 'paints' a baby's digestive tract, stopping harmful microbes getting into his bloodstream. Other fluids or foods can break this barrier-letting infection through.

a day later.[6] In rich societies, the two leading causes of infant death are sudden infant death syndrome (SIDS) and necrotising enterocolitis (NEC).* The risk of a baby suffering these is much lower if they are breastfed. If they are too ill or weak to suckle, they can be fed with expressed breastmilk.

There has never been a single study showing artificial feeding to be better than breastfeeding. So why do whole populations feed their babies manufactured products without an informed understanding of what they do?

Breasts are bad for business

Despite what they say, there is no evidence that the health and wellbeing of infants and mothers is at the heart of what the artificial milk companies do. The spread of artificial feeding is inextricably linked to the growth of commercial milk production, and is a very profitable business. The artificial milk companies' relentless marketing has reached a level where global sales are valued at US$44.8 billion (2014). They are projected to reach US$70.6 billion by 2019.[7]

There is a need for artificial milks. There are still too many orphans and abandoned babies, and too many mothers still die in childbirth.** Women must have the right to breastfeed, but there are still women who don't want to. Why should an individual woman be condemned

---

* For babies with NEC, which affects low birth weight babies who may not be able to suckle, their mother's expressed breastmilk or, as a second best, donated breastmilk, can save their lives.

** Women dying due to complications during pregnancy and childbirth has decreased by 43% from an estimated 532,000 in 1990 to 303,000 in 2015.

for carrying the inhibitions that have been socially and commercially constructed for decades? Ideally, breastmilk banks and wet-nursing should fill all the gaps, but this has not yet been achieved. Then there is the tiny number of women or babies who have a very rare medical problem that makes breastfeeding impossible. Women living with HIV may make an informed decision not to breastfeed or to stop early.[*] A woman whose HIV infection has developed into AIDS should not breastfeed. Most obviously a woman who has had a double mastectomy cannot breastfeed. We need some substitutes for breastmilk, together with the knowledge and skill to use them as safely as possible.

There is actually no perfectly safe way to artificially feed a baby.[**] The products, the equipment and the processes required to make up a feed all introduce the risk of infection. Powdered infant milks can be contaminated with pathogens[***] from the raw ingredients and manufacturing techniques. If these products are not prepared and handled correctly, these pathogens can reproduce to dangerous levels, leading to severe infections that can be fatal. This can happen anywhere in the world.

---

[*] Exclusive breastfeeding in the early months has no higher risk of HIV transmission than exclusive artificial milk feeding. Antiretroviral drugs prevent the transmission of HIV through breastmilk.

[**] See Appendix 2 for how to make up an artificial feed as safely as possible.

[***] These are bacteria and other micro-organisms that can cause disease. *E. Sakazakii* is one of the pathogens found in PIF, and had its name changed to *Cronobacter Sakazakii* in 2007. This has caused infant deaths in rich countries.

Ignorance is not bliss

It's likely that many of you reading this book don't live in extreme poverty, and that you know plenty of artificially fed babies who are alive and kicking. You yourself may not have been optimally breastfed. But babies in rich countries can and do get ill because they are artificially fed, and some die. Where healthcare systems function well, early diagnosis and rapid treatment save lives, but not always. A friend's baby niece, artificially fed from birth, died of pneumonia. Her bereaved parents were expecting another child. I asked if the health professionals had explained to this grieving mother that she could protect her new baby if she breastfed. 'No,' my friend said, 'and I can't tell her and no one else will.' Most of us are afraid of upsetting people so we tiptoe around the truth and betray them as a result.

If you now ask your mother whether she breastfed you and she's upset because she did not, please listen to her story. Forces way beyond her control made it very, very difficult to breastfeed. The same forces still do.

Women who did not breastfeed are often furious with me and the facts. I made mistakes with my children. I crashed the car when they were in the back seat without safety belts. In the 1970s there were no back belts and it was normal to lie your children down unrestrained. Of course I've shuddered at what might have happened. I was following the culture of the time; I did what I thought was OK, but it was not. Thankfully they were fine, but I can't ignore the fact that I might have injured them or worse. Of course I felt guilty but not anymore. Guilt saps your energy and does no good. Toss all guilt out of the window.

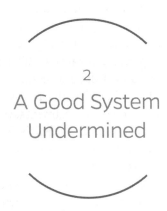

2
A Good System Undermined

Mammals, those creatures that are furry,
warm-blooded, and nourish their young with milk,
are the most popular of all animals – perhaps
because we are mammals ourselves.

David Attenborough

We are mammals

Lactation – making milk – is a fantastic biological strategy and one reason why humans are such a successful species. Because of our large brains we are born too early to survive on our own. We're literally too big-headed for our own good. Unlike most other mammals, baby humans are utterly dependent on their mothers for food and nurture for several years.

For over 90 per cent of human life on earth, there was no milk to replace breastfeeding. If a mother died, another woman breastfed the baby or the baby died. We evolved to thrive on a diet without animal milk. Considering how long humans have been around, milking animals is a very new practice. When human groups started domesticating animals about 10,000 years ago,* milk had to be fermented or soured for it to be digestible. Only mutant northern Europeans (and a few other groups) developed the weird trait of being able to digest lactose (the sugar in milk) after babyhood.**

Since written records began, just over 5,000 years ago, there have been descriptions of feeding animal milk to orphaned babies; sometimes the baby suckled directly from the animal's teat. Most of these babies died.

Ninety per cent of all humans who have ever lived have been gatherer/hunter/foragers. The wild foods around them provided a diverse and nutritious diet. Anyone who studies the few remaining groups who live as our ancestors did finds that breastfeeding 'failure' is unknown to them. Anthropologists James and Lisa Woodburn have known the nomadic Hadza people of Tanzania for over 50 years, and not one Hadza can recall a case of 'not enough' milk or 'failure to breastfeed'. It's the same with Amazonian Indian groups or remote tribes in Papua New Guinea: the suggestion that a woman might not be able to breastfeed provokes astonishment and laughter.

---

* We *Homo sapiens* (wise man) have been around for about 70,000 years, but other humans first evolved 2.5 million years ago.
** This trait is now called alactasia, as though it is an illness, when in fact it has been and is the normal state for most humans.

Women's bodies are amazing

By the 20th century it was commonly believed that poor, underfed women could not provide enough milk for their babies. This idea turned out to be nonsense. Researchers found that rural African women, who endured seasonal hunger, produced just as much milk as overfed Australians and Europeans. Nutrition scientists Ann Prentice and Andrew Prentice added nutrient-rich biscuits to the normal diet of Gambian women and it didn't make a scrap of difference to their breastmilk output.[1] The big factor was the baby. The more a baby suckled, the more breastmilk he stimulated from his mother.

Evidently all women are designed to feed twins, so it is unlikely that a body could not produce enough milk to feed one baby. These are all plain facts. I too was astonished when I learned them. I grew up in the UK where people said 'Are you going to try and breastfeed?' as though you were entering a marathon and would probably have to drop out.

I had an informal training in how breastfeeding worked when I lived in Mozambique in the 1980s. Poverty, hunger and war were everywhere and I just observed mothers and babies. One day Josina came to the clinic to get her five-month-old triplets checked. She was a typical farmer who had five older children who helped with the babies. Josina's triplets were born small,* but had all zoomed up the weight charts and were thriving on breastmilk alone. We European health workers oohed and aahed. Josina did not know what the

---

* Between 2,250g and 2,700g.

fuss was about. She accepted unconsciously what I later learned from formal science: that one baby suckling produced milk, so three babies suckling produced more milk. Indeed, a weaker sibling benefits from the more effective suckling of a stronger sibling, so multiples often help each other. A key factor was that Josina could not get hold of artificial milk because the economic chaos of that time made it unavailable. If she had, her babies might have caught infections, suckled less well and reduced Josina's breastmilk supply.

In the 1980s famine in West Darfur, Sudan, a researcher and campaigner on human rights in Africa, Alex de Waal, looked at the death rates and their causes. He found infant mortality was no different from normal times and realised this was due to exclusive breastfeeding.[2] That's why underfed women in prison camps could keep their babies alive and healthy. Women are more metabolically efficient and can keep going for longer on fewer calories than men.[*] When breastfeeding does go wrong it's usually because the baby has a problem that prevents her from suckling effectively, or she is stopped from doing so. Too many people still don't grasp the basic principle that a woman's breast responds to a baby's behaviour and is not a holding chamber for a

---

[*] Theoretically breastfeeding women need 500kcal extra per day in the first six months. But while this may stave off hunger, it makes no difference to breastmilk supply. Body fat laid down in pregnancy provides a calorie reserve. With pandemic overweight and obesity, even in poor regions, this edict needs re-examining. It may be that the metabolic adaptations of lactation help women conserve energy.

finite supply of milk. As my engineer son summed it up: 'the breast is a gland not a bladder.'

This *does not mean* that women don't have the right to enough good food for their own health. Quite rightly, aid agencies in disasters allow extra food for breastfeeding mothers. A mother needs extra nutrition to regain her strength after the birth and to look after her children but not to make milk. That's the baby's job.

Good men make mistakes

Despite the biological robustness of lactation, we humans are so brilliant at making things complicated and difficult that we could win a gold medal for 'screwing up systems' when it comes to breastfeeding. Let's go back to 18th century England. The great French chemist Louis Pasteur (1822–95), who proved that microbes caused disease, was not yet born. For most of recorded history, birth and breastfeeding were women's business, but then doctors (all male at that time) began to take an interest, for all the right reasons. They wanted to save lives. I'm going to tell you about just one, Dr William Cadogan, because he made such an impact. Other doctors followed in his wake. Through British imperialism, these influential men's ideas spread round the world.

Cadogan had the gift of observation. He noted the frequent deaths of infants. He discovered that ordinary working countrywomen breastfed their babies exclusively from birth. He saw the babies of wealthy families being fed all sorts of ridiculous 'paps and gruels' made of breadcrumbs, wine, butter, cows' milk, water and God knows what else, before they were even put to the breast at all. Also they were usually wet-nursed and there was often a delay in feeding or a change of wet nurse. We might assume that these posh women didn't want to breastfeed, but like most of us they did what families and friends expected of them. Many of these women were not *allowed* to breastfeed. The reason for this will be revealed in the next chapter.

Cadogan kept careful records. When he looked at his data he found that far greater numbers of rich babies died than those of humbler mums. He also found that rich women were more likely to die after childbirth. He realised breastfeeding made the difference.

He published an essay[*] that became a bestseller; it was reprinted several times and widely translated. Cadogan became rich, famous and influential. Because of him it became the trend for posh women to breastfeed their own babies and do so exclusively from birth. Both infant and maternal mortality rates fell. Knowing they were less likely to die after birth motivated rich women to breastfeed, even if it went against their family culture.[**]

Though fashionable and well paid by the rich, Cadogan cared about abandoned and orphaned babies. He organised wet nursing by the sensible countrywomen who breastfed their own children. Like modern foster mothers, they were paid and respected for their skills.

---

[*] Dr William Cadogan, *An Essay upon Nursing and the Management of Children from their Birth to Three Years of Age*, 1748.

[**] Early, exclusive breastfeeding would have helped expel the placenta and would have prevented mastitis. Both these conditions could lead to septicaemia and death.

Most babies lived with them for several years and many lives were saved. In orphanages with no breastfeeding few babies survived. By 1830, the Dublin Foundling Hospital was closed because 99.6 per cent of babies died! One reason was that Catholic wet nurses were forbidden to breastfeed Protestant babies. Likewise, in Austria Christian wet nurses could not feed Jewish babies.

I rather like the idea that religion is passed on through breastmilk. Does this mean that if you are fed on a Danone brand of artificial milk*, you become a devout Danonite? Actually it has been said that Nestlé's promotion of baby milks and baby foods is part of a marketing strategy to create brand loyalty for life, so maybe brand religion is not such a far-fetched idea.

Now for the regrettable bit: Cadogan promoted maternal breastfeeding (wet nursing was second best, but better than no breastfeeding), exclusive breastfeeding from birth and he condemned tight swaddling. This was all good stuff, which modern scientific research backs up as healthy and good. The fact that he recorded and learned from his data was excellent. However, like most popular gurus he made some mistakes and came to some wrong conclusions. He believed, along with other doctors, that 'overfeeding' caused diarrhoea (then, as now, a major killer of babies). In this case, he did not distinguish between breastfeeding and a bowl of mashed bread and cows' milk. Before the invention of fridges, or knowledge of effective hygiene, a lot of food became contaminated.

---

* In 2015 Danone was the second biggest baby milk and baby food manufacturer in the world after Nestlé.

Cadogan could not know that breastmilk contained anti-infective factors. Why should he? The fact that microbes caused disease had not been discovered yet. Restricted feeding had never existed before. He declared that babies should not be breastfed more than five times a day. He did not understand the demand and supply system of lactation. He never suggested limiting the length of a breastfeed – that was left to 20th century doctors – but he did forbid night feeds and sharing the bed with the wet nurse or mother.

I feel fond of Cadogan. He cared about abandoned babies, he scrutinised his data, he got things done. He was quite unaware that one of his rules could do so much damage. I'm afraid to say, in common with many doctors of his time, he had an attitude problem which might put you off him. His essay begins:

> *It is with great pleasure I see at last the preservation of children become the care of men of sense. In my opinion, this business has been too long fatally left to the management of women, who cannot be supposed to have a proper knowledge to fit them for the task, notwithstanding they look upon it as their own province.*[3]

Now let's just see whether a little bit of scheduling does any harm.

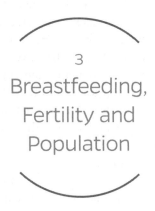

3

Breastfeeding, Fertility and Population

Nature has so wisely ordered things that if women did suckle their children, they would preserve their own health, and there would be such an interval between the birth of each child, that we should seldom see a houseful of babies.

Mary Wollstonecraft (1759–97)*

It didn't work for my mother

Breastfeeding prevents more births worldwide than all other forms of contraception.

'Oh no, that's not true... I'm certain about this because my mother breastfed and her three children were born 13 months apart.'

My challenger, Rowena, is a clever woman; she runs her own business and is a grandmother. I like her. I

---

* Mary Wollstonecraft's book *A Vindication of the Rights of Women* (1792) is seen as the first classic work of feminist thought.

know about this stuff but there's nothing worse than a know-all. In social situations I often bite my tongue, but this time I take courage and plough on:

'Well she did get four months protection then.'

'I suppose so but we all know it doesn't work.'

'Actually it does: there's been good investigation. Researchers found that the !Kung* bushwomen of the Kalahari desert only had children four years apart, but if a baby died at birth they got pregnant again quickly. Unlike in some societies there was no taboo on sex during lactation.'

'So why didn't it work for my mother?'

'Fair question. Because we westerners breastfeed differently. We have schedules, we space out feeds, give water, use dummies and express our milk for someone else to give, and we don't sleep with our babies. To maintain the hormonal state that stops her ovulating, a woman needs to keep her baby close most of the time, especially at night. It's frequent nipple stimulation that stops ovulation, not milk production. The scientists who observed the !Kung mothers and babies noted a suckling episode on average every fourteen minutes.'

'Oh, how dreadful. So you're expecting women to keep their babies permanently attached like leeches? Women aren't going to go back into the box... you can't possibly say...'

Stop right there. When I mention a fact, I am simply telling you a fact. I am not a clergyman delivering a

---

* The exclamation mark represents the 'click' sound in the !Kung language.

sermon. I am not telling you what to do. If I say that prehistoric women breastfed for four to seven years I am not, repeat not, *saying you should do this. When I say gatherer/hunter women provided most of the daily food, consisting of fruits, roots, leaves, little mammals, reptiles and insects, I am not telling you to forage beetles from your local park for the family supper. It's not all about you.*

Of course I didn't say this, because I'm quite polite. I guessed that the bushwomen's contribution to human knowledge was meaningless for Rowena. So I explained about the research with Scottish mothers: as long as their babies suckled at least six times a day, amounting to 65 minutes in total, including some night feeding, they did not ovulate. Suddenly Rowena seemed impressed: Scottish women counted, bushwomen did not.

Cadogan's boob

Now I must explain how our hero of the previous chapter, the excellent William Cadogan, did harm. His advice to restrict the number of breastfeeds to five a day (like daily veg portions – maybe the British just love the number five), and to condemn sleeping with the baby, actually caused a big problem. Cadogan never suggested limiting the length of a feed or time at each breast, as later gurus did, so some babies could stimulate enough milk with just five feeds a day. Many, however, could not, especially in the early weeks, so 'not enough milk' began to be an issue. But the key point here is that the five-a-day babies could not protect their mothers from ovulation. Cadogan's advice lit the fuse of a fertility time bomb.

Getting pregnant too often, or too soon after the previous pregnancy, increases the risk of illness, malnutrition and death for a mother, her toddler and her new baby. If you live in a rich country with good health services you can take this risk, but it's still not ideal. The burden of disease on a society when too many children are born too close together can be profound. The changes in infant feeding practices coincided with rapid population growth. We still can't be sure whether this has been the major cause of population explosions, as there are many other factors, but it has probably made a significant contribution.

When women followed the new health rules and restricted breastfeeding there were more crying babies and more miserable mothers. So what to do? You give the babies other stuff 'in between' feeds. Instead of being offered a breast for food or comfort whenever they asked, babies got water, often mixed with sugar or herbs, called 'bush teas' in the Caribbean.*

From the late 19th century onwards, more and more commercial products flooded on to the market to be the 'stuff in between' breastfeeds. Though the advertising hype boasted of health-giving properties, the nutrient content was far inferior to breastmilk and often harmful.

Giving other foods, fluids or dummies reduces breastmilk supply. By the 20th century women were being told to restrict the minutes a baby spent at the breast and

---

* In the 1970s, my Manchester neighbours advised 'cinder tea': pluck a hot coal from the open fire, put it in water and give the resulting brew to the baby, not forgetting to remove the coal.

to change breasts on the dot of a set time. This created mayhem, as it really did disrupt the essential interaction between a baby and her mother. Clocks and watches were viewed as a key ingredient of infant feeding, yet they interrupted the baby's ability to feed effectively.

Wherever restricting breastfeeding became normal, the problem of 'insufficient milk' spread. The doctors focused on women's failure, as though they could make milk without their babies' suckling. If they didn't have enough milk, it was their fault: they were too sensitive, too red-headed, ate the wrong foods, did not relax and were generally inferior. To this day women blame themselves when breastfeeding goes wrong. And who was waiting in the wings with the expensive substitutes? More of that later, now back to the fertility time bomb.

They bred like rabbits

In many societies in the past people were well aware that breastfeeding prevented pregnancy. Many have condemned the poor for producing too many children, but for centuries it was the rich who bred like rabbits. In much of Europe before the Industrial Revolution, ordinary women controlled their family size through breastfeeding their own and others' babies. That's why aristocratic families used wet nurses. The purpose of a queen or a duchess's life was to produce as many heirs as possible. Posh women had to obey their lords and masters and most were forbidden to breastfeed.

Wealthy 17th-century English heiress Ann Hatton, had 30 children, *'Five sons and eight daughters, besides ten who died young and seven infants stillborn*'. Ordinary women of the day had about seven well-spaced pregnancies at the most. Poor Ann Hatton's life was more like that of a queen termite than a human being. She would not have breastfed any of her children. If we go back to the !Kung bushwomen, or our ancestors who lived similar lives, they had no contraception or taboos against sex soon after birth. Protected by breastfeeding, they had no more than six children in a lifetime and of course fewer miscarriages.

Only exceptional noblewomen breastfed their children. In 13th century France, Blanche of Castile, mother of King Louis IV, was so committed to maternal breastfeeding that when a lady-in-waiting breastfed little Louis when he cried (a common practice; they longed for the honour of suckling a prince), she made him vomit up the milk. This was so remarkable it was documented.

Slavery

If you have seen the Steve McQueen film *Twelve Years a Slave* you will have a vision[*] of one of the worst examples of humanity's cruelty to humanity. The control of women's reproduction was one of many abuses. Slavery had existed for centuries, but as the European colonies expanded so did the slave trade. The wealth, created during the 18th and 19th centuries of the Industrial Revolution in Europe, was based on cheap raw materials such as cotton and sugar; cheap because they were

---

[*] Extreme and sadistic punishments were routinely used for the most trivial matters.

produced by slave labour.

After a phase of 'discouraging' slaves from bearing children, just letting them die and importing more from Africa, slave breeding began to interest the plantation managers. In 19th century Jamaica a Dr Williamson, with the professional detachment of a pig farmer, found it more efficient to breed slaves than continually replace them with newly transported ones, *because a more vigorous set of labourers than the Africans generally become was brought forward in the course of time*. So marriage was promoted and inducements were offered to women to bear children. Women were excused certain tasks and given more free time for each child reared past infancy. The babies were breastfed, but kept in nurseries during working hours. Mothers were allowed two one-hour periods for breastfeeding. If the babies needed food in between they were given 'panada', a mixture of bread, flour and sugar. Mothers were forbidden to breastfeed after 16 months and were separated from their children.

In 1811 Dr Collins wrote his *Practical Rules for the Management and Medical Treatment of Negro Slaves in the Sugar Colonies:*[1]

> *Negroes are universally fond of suckling their children for a long time. If you permit them they will extend it to the third year... Their motives for this are habit, an idea of its necessity, the desire of being spared at their labour or perhaps the avoiding of another pregnancy; but from whichever of these motives they do it your business is to counteract*

their designs and to oblige them to wean their
children as soon as they have attained their 14th or
16th month… If you neglect to do this, you not only
lose some of the mother's labour but you prevent
their breeding so soon.

When you've stopped gasping at this brutality, you might ask how the contraceptive effect worked if the babies were given 'panada' and the women had to restrict daytime feeds. Well, here are some more facts.

The clever system

On average, women who breastfeed ovulate 40 weeks after birth* and women who don't breastfeed at all 11 weeks after birth. As explained earlier, this clever hormonal system works if the baby breastfeeds frequently, including some night feeding. If the baby is fed the mother's expressed breastmilk in a bottle or cup the system fails; it's the nipple stimulation that controls the hormones. How does a woman know whether she's ovulating or not? Breastfeeding women don't have menstrual periods, a liberating experience that protects them from iron-deficiency anaemia and saves money and discomfort. When babies get older and start to eat solid food and suckle less, some women will have a period – a warning sign of returning fertility. However, a tiny number of women might ovulate before this first period and they are at risk of pregnancy.

---

* This is if the woman continues to breastfeed. Whenever a woman stops breastfeeding the likelihood of ovulation returns.

The Lactational Amenorrhoea Method (LAM)[2]*
A woman can use LAM as a method of contraception if:
1. Her menstrual periods have not returned since childbirth.
2. Breastfeeding is baby-led day and night, and breastfeeds are not replaced with other foods or liquids.
3. Her baby is less than six months old.

This method of birth control has a 98 per cent efficacy rate, more reliable than diaphragms or condoms, during the first six months after birth. Though reliability decreases after six months, it can and does go on working for months and even years.

Some women stop breastfeeding because they want another child. Those slave women in 19th century Jamaica slept with their babies. Most mothers in history have done this, because there were no separate rooms and the family would not sleep if the baby cried all night (still the case today for most human beings).

Continued night breastfeeding delayed ovulation. Slave manager Dr Williamson knew this, so he put a stop to it. In the 21st century financial profits continue to be a higher priority than young children's emotional well-being. I can't even broach the topic of emotional damage to babies, because it would take another chapter.

You could say: 'What's this 'breastfeeding as a

---

* Amenorrhoea is the medical term for the absence of menstrual periods. The spelling problem alone echoes how difficult women's lives can be.

contraceptive' malarkey got to do with me? Why can't they just dole out contraceptives to these women?' If only it were that easy. The very fact you have access to this book makes you a privileged person. I want everyone to have access to effective and safe contraception, to knowledge about safe sex and different ways of making love; most of all I want women only to have sex when they want it.

However, right now there are 220 million women in the world who don't want to get pregnant and have no access to contraception and family planning services. Less than a fifth of women in sub-Saharan Africa and barely a third in South Asia use modern contraception. Where can they get it? Where is the clinic? Where are the trained staff? Who provides the money to pay for these services? In 2012, an estimated 80 million women in poor countries got pregnant when they did not want to. At least one in four resorted to unsafe abortion.

Dr William Cadogan and his followers' commands to limit the frequency of breastfeeding and stop night feeding changed the fundamental fertility patterns that 'nature had so wisely ordered'. Though enthusiastic about the life-saving importance of breastfeeding, this mistaken idea is likely to have contributed to the explosion of the fertility time bomb. The harm of closely spaced pregnancies and too rapid population growth cannot be underestimated. Poor old Cadogan: he did so much good and so much harm and was quite unaware of the consequences.

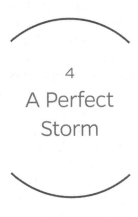

4

A Perfect Storm

*We're very good at inventing things but
very bad at dealing with the consequences.*

Yuval Noah Harari

Tradition is not always best

Please don't think that the past was all rosy. Societies,
old and new, have irrational practices embedded in
their cultures. An astonishing array of interventions
have been judged essential for babies: smacking them
at birth, poking 'symbolic' foods like honey into their
newborn mouths, piercing their ears, snipping their
genitals and tight swaddling are just a few. Despite these
follies, women have always known how to breastfeed. It
was a daily normality throughout their lives.

Look at how modern toddlers can seize your
smartphone and even connect before you think they're
capable. Few children have a crisis of confidence

with modern technology. They've grown up seeing everyone using it and have absorbed the techniques unconsciously. We all know that in communities where everyone dances, no one needs a leaflet or a special tutor to learn how to dance. If you grow up seeing babies feeding from their mothers' breasts, you don't perceive it as problematic. You don't even think about it. You just do it. The researchers in the Gambia (see chapter 2) only ever met one woman with breastfeeding problems and she had, unusually, given birth in hospital.

During the 20th century breastfeeding declined and problems increased wherever hospital births became the norm, but practices are not always ideal with home births. In rural Ghana, where most babies were born at home, Dr Karen Edmunds that found a high number of infant deaths were due to delayed breastfeeding.[1] Karen discovered that mothers waited several hours or even days before the first feed. When she explained the importance of breastfeeding immediately after birth, there was a revolution in practice and infant death rates plummeted.

Now let's get back to the 19th century when many of women's unconscious skills and knowledge of breastfeeding were blown out of existence by the perfect storm of commercial interests and medical beliefs.

The creation of a market

Cows' milk has been the commonest substitute for breastmilk, not because it's the best, but because it's the most available. It still is. Improved dairy farming in the

19th century led to a surplus of cows' milk. Engineers invented techniques of milk preservation. Industrial methods such as roller drying and condensation produced large quantities of powdered and condensed milk. Wherever there is an abundance of a raw material and a new manufacturing process, there is a twinkle in a businessman's eye.* Then he must create the market. As famous business guru Peter Drucker (1909–2005) said: '*Markets are not created by God… it's business action that creates the customer.*' [2]

Dairy cows have been bred to produce far more milk than any calf needs; indeed, it would kill a calf to ingest all of his modern mother's daily supply. Gorillas' milk might be a more suitable breastmilk substitute, but it's impossible to collect. Even with the latest scientific techniques, substitutes for breastmilk are still the palest of imitations.

Cows' milk is still cheap and plentiful. In most industrialised countries, including the USA and Europe, production has been subsidised for decades. The artificial milk companies' huge profits are in part due to taxpayers' support. We pay twice to make them rich. Among the wealthy nations today, only New Zealand and Australia have ended direct dairy subsidies. In the USA, the dairy industry has been such a generous donor to political campaign funds that, despite pushing free market policies on the whole world, no US government has yet dared to end subsidies.

---

* Yes, I know there are businesswomen too, but in those days they were all men.

Get the marketing message right

In 1867, grain and fertiliser merchant Henri Nestlé launched his *farine lactée*, a mixture of wheat flour and condensed milk, with a brilliant promotional puff. He announced that his product had saved the life of *le petit Wanner*, a premature baby who had 'rejected his mother's milk and all other food'. By 15 days, little Wanner had convulsions and hope for his life was fading. Then Henri Nestlé came to the rescue with his *farine lactée*. By seven months, little Wanner, fed exclusively on Nestlé's *farine,* had never been ill and could sit up alone in his cradle.

Within five years, Nestlé was selling half a million boxes of *farine lactée* a year in Europe, the USA, Latin America, Australia and the Dutch East Indies. There's a strong health message here, for business health that is: it doesn't matter how nutritionally inadequate your product is, get your PR message perfect and you're in. Be the first in the market and you'll be market leader over a century later.

I always wondered why 'little Wanner' was not wet-nursed,[*] a normal practice in those days; perhaps he was the wrong religion. As for exclusive feeding with a wheat flour and condensed milk[**] mixture for the first seven months – nowadays his parents would be charged with neglect. It just shows how tough some babies are. Or perhaps, along with all promotional copy, we must take Henri Nestlé's claim with a big pinch of salt.

---

[*] Or fed a wet nurse's expressed milk.
[**] Condensed milk lacked vitamins A and D.

Nestlé was soon market leader and setting promotional trends. Throughout the 19th century, a variety of milks and foods for infants, as well as bottles and teats, were widely promoted. Doctors had no idea how to help women with breastfeeding difficulties. In France, the well-intentioned Dr Pierre Budin (1846–1907) strongly approved of breastfeeding, but accepted 'failure' as incurable. He shared the now well-established horror of 'overfeeding'. He set up 'milk depots' to provide uncontaminated cows' milk at a lowish price for mothers judged unable to breastfeed.

This idea spread to Holland, Britain, North America, Australia and New Zealand. Some claimed these milk depots saved lives, but in 1917 the *British Medical Journal* found no difference in infant death rates between towns with or without milk depots. The majority of the population had neither fridges nor indoor plumbing, and keeping even sterilised milk clean and safe was impossible.[*] Artificially fed babies died in large numbers in both Europe and the USA. What the milk depots did was to establish a link between the supervision of mothers and babies by health professionals and the distribution of substitutes for breastfeeding.

Milk and murder

Early attempts at regulating the advertising of infant foods first occurred in Britain and then in the USA. In Britain, Dr Coutts' 1911 *Report on the Unsuitability of*

---

[*]   In contrast, breastmilk can be kept at room temperature for six hours, in a fridge at 0–4°C for eight days and in the freezer at −18°C or lower for six months. (Source: Breastfeeding Network).

Sweetened Condensed Milk (SCM)[3] as an infant food was discussed in Parliament. SCM was condemned and conspicuous labelling demanded. In what was to become a long-term game, companies exploited loopholes to get round laws. Regulation required SCM labels to state *'unsuitable for infants'*. One label put this in tiny print, but claimed in huge letters: 'FOR INFANTS AND INVALIDS'. Manufacturers boasted of 'purity' and 'sterility', but most brands tested in Dr Coutts' report contained pathogens.

While the dangers of SCM and other artificial milks were being tackled in the 'mother country', marketing continued in the colonies. In Malaysia,* newspapers advertised milks for infants from the 1880s onwards. By the 1920s, 18 brands featured in 30 to 40 ads a month together with bottle and teat promotion. While British colonial nurses tut-tutted at breastfeeding on demand and pushed clocks, bottles and strict schedules at local mothers, Nestlé advertised SCM to doctors as *'…the food par excellence for delicate infants'.**

This cynical promotion prompted the famous paediatrician, Dr Cicely Williams, to call her 1939 speech to the Singapore Rotary Club 'Milk and Murder', in which she said *'…if your lives were embittered as mine is, by seeing day after day this massacre of the innocents by unsuitable feeding, then I would believe you would feel as I do that misguided propaganda on infant feeding should be punished as the most miserable form of sedition*

---

* Called Malaya by the British Colonial administrators.
** As claimed a Nestlé diary for doctors in 1936.

and that these deaths should be regarded as murder.[4] The club's chairman was the president of Nestlé.

The International Baby Food Action Network (IBFAN) considers Dr Cicely Williams (1893–1992) to be the founder of the campaign to stop the immoral marketing of infant feeding products.

During the Second World War, Cicely Williams was imprisoned in Japanese internment camps in Singapore. Among many things, she taught me that mothers could breastfeed in the worst conditions when she described the '*twenty babies born, twenty babies breastfed, twenty babies grew up healthy,*' of the British women imprisoned with her.

Now perhaps to the most destructive blast of the perfect storm.

A very happy marriage

You may have noticed that I try to avoid the word 'infant formula'. This is because it is a marketing term, coined by US doctors at the turn of the 19th and 20th centuries.[*] The doctors persuaded mothers that artificial feeding was 'scientific', experimenting with recipes for individual babies and convincing mothers to return (and pay) each week for minor adjustments to a concoction made up in a back room. To add mystique to this service, doctors presented their recipes as algebraic formulas to impress mothers. A cake is a mixture of ingredients, and if you presented these in algebraic terms you could call a cake,

---

* In 1911, 58% of US babies were breastfed at 12 months. Thereafter it was a steady decline in incidence and duration of breastfeeding until the 1970s.

$$M = \frac{Qb - bC}{b} \quad C = \frac{L(b^1 F - a^1 P)}{ab^1 - a^1 b} \quad C = (2F + S + P) \times 1\tfrac{1}{4} Q$$

Early 20th century example of formula used for calculating a baby's artificial feed.[5]

'formula'. The fact that a trick term to describe a basic mixture of cows' milk, sugar and water is now used in official regulatory documents shows how influential a marketing term can be.

While the US doctors insisted on custom-made preparations for their wealthy patients, poorer mothers were buying commercial milks, widely advertised as safe and superior. The doctors protested because they lost income and prestige. In 1893 the influential Dr Thomas Morgan Rotch wrote:

> *The proper authority for establishing rules for substitute feeding should emanate from the medical profession, and not from the non-medical capitalists.*

But the mothers carried on buying the products. Advertising works.

The manufacturers soon realised that conflict did not serve their interests. They began to woo the doctors, who were tired of fiddling about with milk and sugar in their surgeries. One doctor did a deal with an infant food manufacturer, Mead Johnson, who made up his favourite recipe and tested it on babies in the New York Post-Graduate Hospital in 1911. No problems with ethical committees then. The manufacturers and the doctors became friendlier. The ads in the popular press began to direct the consumer to a doctor and the ads in the medical journals praised the ease of preparation that *'rouses the parents' enthusiasm and adds to the prestige of the physician.'* That poor mothers could not afford both the product and a doctor's fee did not seem to bother either the manufacturers or the doctors.

Some doctors, especially those confronting the frequent illnesses and deaths of artificially fed babies, were concerned about the negative effect on breastfeeding of widespread advertising. In 1924, the American Medical Association set up a committee of investigation. The results moved the friendship between the companies and the medical profession into a love affair that blossomed into the happy marriage that lasts to this day. The most honest statement about this period comes from Mead Johnson:

> *When mothers in America feed their babies by lay advice, the control of your pediatric cases passes out of your hands, Doctor. Our interest in this important phase of medical economics springs, not from any motives of altruism, philanthropy or paternalism, but rather from a spirit of enlightened self interest and cooperation because [our] infant diet materials are advertised only to you, never to the public.*[6]

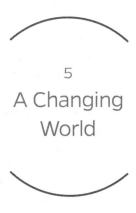

5
A Changing World

There is no finer investment for any community than putting milk into babies.

Winston Churchill (1874–1965)

Hospital habits

By the end of the Second World War (1945) artificial feeding was becoming normal in the industrialised world. Rich women, who once hired wet nurses, could now buy a modern 'scientific product'. Many saw these man-made milks as superior to breastmilk. A lot of doctors and midwives noticed the lower rates of disease in breastfed babies, but by now breastfeeding failure was accepted as a common flaw of women's bodies, or even a defect of female willpower. People were led to believe that many women could not produce enough milk and that breastfeeding often needed to be supplemented.

Established with the best of intentions, hospital

practices sabotaged easy breastfeeding, turning a joyful bonding into a nightmare. Babies were separated at birth, kept in nurseries and given sugar water* or artificial milks. Before the invention of 'ready to feed' milks in individual bottles, most maternity wards had a 'milk kitchen' where nurses and midwives wasted hours making up artificial feeds while babies screamed in the nursery and their mothers lay bemused in their beds.

Health staff brought the babies to the mothers at 'feed times'. Mothers were told to wash their nipples before and after every breastfeed. They were told to wait for their milk to 'come in' as though the baby had nothing to do with the process. Sore nipples were believed to be the result of too much – rather than poorly attached – suckling. Supplementary bottles of artificial milk were brought with the babies and sat menacingly on the bedside table to be used as 'top ups' after a mother had given her baby a brief and strictly timed session at each breast. Babies were test-weighed before and after breastfeeds. If they were judged not to have taken in enough breastmilk, mothers were blamed: 'Your nipples are too flat; you're not relaxed enough; you must persist.' The list of female inadequacy was never ending. 'Why didn't they consider the baby's role?', I hear you cry. They didn't know or notice.

Until 2006, WHO child growth standards were based on US babies who were mostly artificially fed and grew rather big rather quickly. Mothers around the world were

---

* Glucose and dextrose are no different from regular sugar (sucrose) in the effect they have on a baby's feeding.

told they did not have enough breastmilk to keep their babies growing. Then WHO monitored the growth of 8,000 breastfed children in six different countries. Over 15 years, using the best methods, they discovered that babies were not meant to grow that fast or get that heavy. The breastfed babies, the 'gold standard', were longer and leaner. They had different metabolic rates and sleeping patterns and they self-regulated their food intake. WHO had to create new growth standards and the artificial milks had to be reformulated to do less harm. Excess weight gain is now a global pandemic causing long-term health problems such as diabetes and heart disease, and it starts in infancy. Breastfeeding protects against obesity.

With strict schedules and no skin contact, mothers had little chance to get to know their babies, who were whisked away to the hospital nurseries between feeds. Many health professionals could not recognise a baby's feeding cues,* or help a mother hold her baby comfortably and help him suckle effectively.

Way back in 1903, leading US physician Dr Koplik had written, *'The thumb may be used to exert pressure on the breast, thus aiding the flow of milk. In this way the infant is prevented from drawing the nipple too far*

---

* Turning their heads, protruding their tongues, pushing their fists into their mouths. When these cues are ignored and babies have to scream with hunger to get fed, feeding difficulties are more common.

into the mouth.' Good, caring Dr Koplik, who provided free sterilised cows' milk for poor New York women, completely misunderstood breastfeeding. The flow is not 'aided by pressure', but triggered by the 'hormone of love',* oxytocin, which ejects the milk in response to the suckling action of a baby's mouth. Effective 'attachment' at the breast (key to breastfeeding) depends on the baby drawing the nipple far back into her mouth. Engorgement, sore nipples, breast abscesses, mastitis and insufficient milk became common as women, grievously misinformed, did as they were told. No wonder mothers told their daughters not to bother with this horrible experience.

The unwitting suppression

By the 1950s, it had become normal to give routine lactation suppressants after birth in US maternity wards and the practice spread to Europe. The majority of North American babies were artificially fed either with commercial 'infant formulas' or homemade dilutions of fresh, evaporated or condensed milk. By the 1970s, in much of Europe breastfeeding was neglected and gradually abandoned as artificial milks became widely available, often provided cheaply or free by governments. Meanwhile, in most of the world, breastfeeding was still the norm but rapidly being undermined.

In the aftermath of the Second World War, UNICEF and other agencies distributed milk for children worldwide. Though done in good faith, the distribution of milk had a

---

* The obstetrician Michel Odent calls oxytocin 'the hormone of love'.

devastating effect on breastfeeding. It unwittingly created a link between children's health and cows' milk. Western ideals of nutrition and dairy-centric diets were being imposed onto societies without considering the possible damage. Many people perceived this milk as a substitute for breastfeeding, and the fact that high status agencies distributed it made it appear essential. This substitution went hand in hand with health messages to discourage breastfeeding after one year.

In the UK, the well-organised public health and food distribution system of the Second World War[*] had introduced state-subsidised National Dried Milk as a breastmilk substitute for those women considered unable to breastfeed. When British prime minister Winston Churchill declared that there was no finer investment than putting milk into babies he tactfully endorsed both breastfeeding and artificial feeding as equal. Most people thought they were. Commerce was not the only cause of the problem.

Why did they not all die?

In the industrialised countries health was improving and child death rates were falling, despite the increase in artificial feeding. Twentieth century public health measures such as safe, piped water and a toilet in every home, public sewers and better housing with reduced overcrowding changed people's lives. Such improved

---

[*] Britain won the US Lasker Prize for its excellence in public health during and after WW2. Health indicators had never improved so fast or so successfully.

living standards had a marked effect on health; for example, that's why tuberculosis (TB) rates fell long before effective TB drugs were widely available. These improvements, together with adequate food supplies and access to healthcare, created a child survival revolution.

Immunisation cancelled out previously inevitable deaths from measles, diphtheria, polio and other infections. Education and literacy meant that families could read instructions and sterilise infant feeding equipment. Health visitors, midwives and public health nurses recognised early signs of illness and could judge when to consult a doctor. In 1948 the UK's newly formed National Health Service meant families need not worry about treatment costs and most industrialised countries established free or affordable healthcare for mothers and babies. This environment significantly lowered the risks and masked the impact of not breastfeeding.

Selling to the shack

The second half of the 20th century saw huge political, social and economic changes. As the dust settled after the Second World War, business looked to the future. The colonised nations in Africa and Asia demanded political independence and, after struggles and bloody conflict, won it. There was business optimism as big companies envisaged high profits from these emerging markets. Nestlé already had its foot in the door. It had been marketing artificial milks globally since the late 19th century and now new techniques were turning the art of promotion into a science.

Radio sets had spread across the world, so promotion could reach the illiterate, including the majority of women in Africa. In one month in 1974 in Sierra Leone, 135 ads for Nestlé's Lactogen were broadcast in the local language. In another, 45 ads for Cow & Gate baby milks and 66 for Abbott-Ross' Similac were aired. Nestlé proclaimed in Creole: *'Now Lactogen a better food cos it don get more protein and iron, all the important things dat go make pikin strong and well. Lactogen Full Protein now get more cream taste and Nestlé den guarantee um… Lactogen and Love.'* Ironically, more protein and iron are dangerous for an infant's health.

Company research found that *'Depth interviews brought out very clearly the mothers' positive attitude to bottlefeeding.'* [1]

Mothers were convinced that artificial milk was a medicine, especially as it was promoted in health clinics and maternity wards. Most saw it as a bonus to enhance a baby's health. None of this promotion mentioned the risks, even though they quickly became apparent.

Milk company staff were well aware that the rural villages, shanty towns and growing slums lacked clean running water, sanitation and literacy. All the companies behaved unethically, but market leader Nestlé set the trends:

> *The advent of television as a universal means of communicating with the shack as well as the mansion permits the standardisation to an increasing extent of advertising and promotion.*

Nestlé uses the medium extensively wherever it can. Where it still can't, the company relies on newspapers, colour magazines, billboards and outdoor displays. In less developed countries, the best form of promoting baby food formulas may well be the clinics which the company sponsors, at which nurses and doctors in its employ offer childcare guidance service... effective distribution may call for unusual, imaginative techniques.[2]

One imaginative technique was the use of 'milk nurses' – saleswomen dressed in nurses' uniforms – adding medical prestige to their sales pitch. Dr Cicely Williams described them as '*dragging a good lactating breast out of the baby's mouth and pouring in baby milks*'.[3]

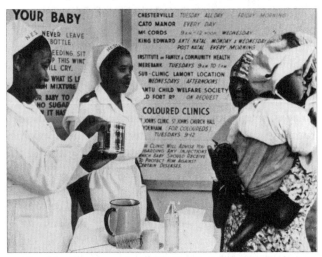

Nestlé milk nurses in 1950s South Africa (photo Nestlé in Profile)

Commerciogenic malnutrition

By the 1950s and 60s doctors working in Africa and Asia had already been alarmed by the increasing number of young babies brought to clinics with severe diarrhoea and malnutrition. Traditionally mothers breastfed each child for two or three years. In the first year a baby could thrive on breastmilk alone, but as inadequate or contaminated foods gradually replaced breastfeeding, a cycle of infection and malnutrition set in causing many deaths. The doctors had rarely seen malnutrition in such young babies; now they were seeing it frequently. They discovered that mothers were bottlefeeding artificial milks. The doctors called this condition 'commerciogenic malnutrition' or 'bottle baby disease'.

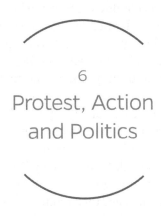

6
Protest, Action and Politics

Whose responsibility is it to control the advertising, marketing and promotional activities which may create a market in spite of public health considerations?

Edward Kennedy (1932–2009)

A mother and her daughter

In 1970, Wangari was living on the edge of Nairobi in a two-room, wood and cane house with a corrugated zinc roof. It was often over 40°C inside, but Wangari was used to it. Her four-year-old son was thriving and she was delighted when she gave birth to a healthy daughter, not yet named for fear of ill fortune. Wangari was pleased when the milk nurses came to town and explained that she could buy the milks the rich, white women fed their babies. Of course she was breastfeeding; she'd never considered anything else, or known anyone who had not, but babies could get ill and this special milk, advertised daily on the radio, would provide extra protection. The friendly nurses showed how to mix the powdered milk with water and even gave her a free tin to take home. Her husband told her not to trust these white men's things, but she dismissed his old fashioned ideas.

Borrowing the money from her sister, she bought a bottle and teat from a store. Like all her neighbours, Wangari fetched her water from a pool half a mile away, carrying the 20 litre metal can home on her head. Neighbours did this for her in the weeks after the birth, but she was back to normal now her daughter was three months old and growing well. Wangari couldn't read the label, but she recalled exactly how the nurse made up the artificial milk. She fed it to her daughter in the bottle and felt proud.

Some days later her baby was feverish and had diarrhoea. Perhaps more of the special milk would help? That evening she fed her daughter half of a full bottle of milk and saved the rest overnight, carefully covered with a cloth in case of insects. Wangari carried on breastfeeding but, as the diarrhoea continued, her baby grew weaker and more fretful and seemed to lose the strength to suckle. Soon the powdered milk began to run out, so she added a bit more water to the mix. Over the next few days, when she breastfed her miserable, crying daughter, she sensed there was not the usual copious flow of milk. Her first thought was that someone had put a curse on her. Her second was that she must buy more powdered milk, but she hadn't enough money. What should she do?

Her baby now had dark shadows round her eyes, was visibly thinner and her skin was saggy. Wangari left her son with a neighbour, tied her daughter on her back and went to her sister's house. On her sister's advice, they walked the three miles in the hot sun to the nearest hospital. She tried to breastfeed during the journey but her daughter was too weak to suckle. When they arrived, they had to wait in the queue. The doctors put her baby on an intravenous drip to treat the dehydration caused by the gastrointestinal infection she had taken in with her artificial milk feed.

Whistleblowers, doctors and the UN

The doctors working in that African hospital, and in other regions where poverty was normal, were becoming aware of the harm of artificial milk promotion. Some tried to stop it. In Nigeria, Dutch paediatrician Catherine Wennen, struggling to save the lives of babies like Wangari's, noticed the closeness between the companies' managers and the elite doctors who happily accepted gifts for their hospitals and themselves. She contacted the Nestlé manager in Lagos to explain the problem, but he didn't want to listen.

Since the mid-1960s, health professionals had been writing to the biggest milk supplier, Nestlé, to explain the dangers of artificial feeding in poor communities. Their letters were ignored unless bad publicity threatened. A young scientist working in Jamaica, Ann Ashworth Hill, alerted Nestlé to the misinformation on the Sweetened Condensed Milk labels – still there

50 years after condemnation by the British government. Ann was researching ways to save the lives of Jamaican babies suffering the same cycle of infection and malnutrition that Wangari's daughter suffered. Nothing happened. Then Ann's husband, Jamaican MP Winston Hill, asked questions in the Jamaican Parliament. Immediately Nestlé executives flew in, listened to Ann, and changed the labels… in Jamaica.

By 1970 the UN was involved, but meetings of UN officials, health professionals and representatives of the baby food industry achieved nothing. Then in 1974 some timely journalism highlighted the issue through the world's media. Paediatrician Dr Derrick Jelliffe, working in Africa and the Caribbean, published an article called 'Commerciogenic Malnutrition'.[1] The magazine *New Internationalist* interviewed two respected paediatricians, David Morley and Ralph Hendrikse, who starkly described the suffering and deaths. Finally, the UK charity War on Want brought out *The Baby Killer*, a booklet describing

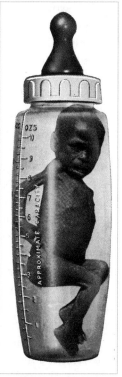

Graphic used on the front cover of *The Baby Killer* by Mike Muller 1974 (War on Want).

in clear words and pictures the tragic effects of baby milk promotion in the real living conditions of most of humanity.[2] The front cover caused a sensation, 20,000 copies quickly sold and it was widely translated.

The Nestlé trial

One translation caused a firestorm. A Swiss action group[*] called its German version *Nestlé Tötet Babys...* 'Nestlé Kills Babies'. Nestlé[**] sued the group and won. This sounds bad, but in fact the lawsuit raised more awareness than the booklet itself. Nestlé at first charged the group on four counts of libel: the title; the accusations of unethical practices; responsibility for death or damage to babies; and dressing saleswomen as nurses. By the final court hearing Nestlé had withdrawn all charges except for the title. The judge ruled this libellous because members of the Nestlé company had not actually killed babies; the mothers had done the killing when they bottlefed them with the artificial milks.

Don't hate the judge. He used his authority to give Nestlé a fierce and humiliating telling-off. The witnesses throughout the hearings, including several highly respected doctors,[***] had exposed the trickery and ruthlessness of Nestlé and educated the press and the public about the effects of unregulated marketing on infant health and survival. People were shocked. The

---

[*]   Arbeitsgruppe Dritte Welt (AgDW)

[**] Nestlé had iconic status in Switzerland and was the biggest food company in the world.

[***] One of the doctors was Dr Zef Ebrahim, to whom this book is dedicated.

judge stated: *'If the complainant in future wants to be spared the accusation of immoral and unethical conduct, he will have to change advertising practices.'* The Swiss group was given a token fine.

It's important to emphasise that other baby food companies behaved badly too, but their smaller market share meant they damaged fewer babies. At that time Nestlé supplied at least three-quarters of the global market and, as they themselves boasted, led the world in innovative marketing techniques. In the USA, a group of Catholic nuns[*] had, as shareholders, sued Bristol Myers for their immoral marketing of artificial milks in Central America. The judge dismissed the case because the nuns themselves had not suffered harm. When the nuns appealed, Bristol Myers settled out of court, but again the publicity raised awareness of the issue.

The Nestlé boycott

Despite the lawsuits, the Swiss judge's humiliating statements and the bad press coverage, Nestlé's promotion and sales continued. By now activists were gathering and asking each other what could be done. A catalyst was Peter Krieg's 1975 film, *Bottle Babies*. When viewers saw a mother scooping water from a dirty pool, and a malnourished baby screaming as health workers struggled to get a drip needle into a head vein, the pain they had read about was brought to life. Inspired by the film, a group of energetic young men and women in the USA launched The Infant Formula Action Group

---

[*] 1975 The Sisters of the Precious Blood.

(INFACT). They publicly announced a boycott of Nestlé food products,* urging people to join. Their goal was to pressure Nestlé into stopping the promotion of artificial milk, particularly through milk nurses, free samples and direct advertising. The boycott spread to Canada, Europe, Australia and New Zealand.

In the USA, Nestlé sales started to fall. Instead of changing its practices, Nestlé paid US$1 million (US$4 million today) to a PR company to target US clergy with glossy booklets boasting that the company did not engage in unethical promotion. This alerted many churches to the issue and they joined the movement, some gathering fresh evidence from their overseas missionaries. By late 1977, health professionals, women's and students' groups, trade unions, celebrities and prominent politicians were involved in the boycott.

Another of Nestlé's PR advisors proposed a withdrawal from the infant food market, arguing that as a proportion of all their product sales, infant milk profits were not worth the reputational damage. Was corporate pride stronger than corporate greed? The internal arguments within Nestlé may never come to light, but what is on record is the involvement of the US Government.

Power and influence

Most people see the USA as a leader in business deregulation. In the 1980s, during the Reagan presidency,

---

* The boycotters did not include Nestlé infant milks in the boycott because in some places it was the only breastmilk substitute on the market; they did not want to jeopardise an artificially fed baby's nutrition.

the famous Chicago School of neoliberal economic theory preached that the less regulated corporations were, the richer and happier the world would be. British prime minister Margaret Thatcher backed this philosophy and more and more countries were converted to these ideas. It is easy to forget that the USA had a long-established tradition of action to restrict the harm companies could inflict. The 1890 Sherman Anti-trust Act outlawed cartels, monopolies, price fixing, inferior goods and services and the suppression of competition and innovation. It was probably this old proud spirit of justice that in 1978 inspired US Senator Edward Kennedy* to set up the Official Hearing into the global marketing of infant milks.

Kennedy's Hearing exposed more appalling practices that revealed just how cold-blooded the company leaders were. Nestlé became ever more defensive, taking the line that the activists were, *'Marxists marching under the banner of Christ'*. This made many a nun laugh. Kennedy realised that the USA alone could not solve the problem. A global effort was needed and the WHO and UNICEF were the right bodies to create an 'International Code of Marketing of Breastmilk Substitutes' (the Code). This would create a level playing field for the whole infant food industry. Meetings were set up between WHO and UNICEF bureaucrats, the infant food industry representative body,** the health experts, the activists and lawyers for all sides and they got down to the business of creating the Code. This brief explanantion oversimplifies

---

* In his role as Chair of the Senate Sub-Committee on Health and Scientific Research.

** International Council of Infant Food Industries (ICIFI).

The basics of 'the Code' and later resolutions on infant and young child feeding:

1. No public promotion of breastmilk substitutes in any form. (This includes bottles and teats.)
2. No promotion in health facilities or to health workers.
3. No free or low cost supplies.
4. All information for health professionals about breastmilk substitutes must be scientific and factual (no promotional content).
5. Product labels must have full, clear information, correct instructions for safe use and no baby pictures or idealising images or language.
6. All products must be of high quality and conform to Codex* quality and safety standards.
7. Companies to comply with the Code even if a government does not.
8. Promotion of complementary foods must not undermine breastfeeding.
9. Governments are responsible for providing clear, consistent and impartial information on infant feeding.
10. Governments to avoid conflicts of interest.

* see note page 65

the complex political dynamics and conflicting agendas which made the process far more difficult than we could ever imagine.

After over two years of hard work, with all the inevitable wrangling and compromises, agreement was reached and the Code was ready. In 1981 it was adopted at the World Health Assembly (WHA)* by an overwhelming majority of votes. There were three abstentions and one single vote against. Why am I bothering to tell you this? Well, that 'no' vote came from the USA. Other countries with strong free market ideologies (and baby food industries), including Margaret Thatcher's UK, supported this international effort to protect all infants.

The irony was that the nation whose people had protested most passionately, whose government had investigated the issue most thoroughly, and who had launched the very concept of the Code, had just voted in President Reagan, who was to undermine it. This had little to do with Nestlé. It was the US infant food companies who had lobbied Reagan and persuaded him to undo the good work that his country had done for global child survival.

The two chief delegates for the US Government, who had worked so hard to achieve a moderate Code acceptable to US ideas of business practice, were ordered the night before the vote to reverse their stance. These two men returned to the USA from the WHO in Geneva and resigned from their jobs.

The Code was adopted by an overwhelming majority, but without one of the most powerful players.**

And what about Wangari and her baby? Wangari's daughter died without a name.

---

* The World Health Assembly represents 'we the people' and makes decisions about global health issues. The WHO is supposed to implement these decisions.
** The USA signed up to the Code in a 1994 World Health Assembly (WHA) Resolution, but they have done little to implement it.

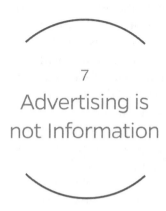

7

Advertising is not Information

If advertising simply provided information, it would be hard to object. But a lot of advertising makes us feel we need something that previously we didn't need.

Richard Layard

An everyday advert

I'm addicted to crosswords; I'm stuck so I search a website to check a word. As usual an advert pops up on the screen and this time it's for *'Aptamil with Pronutra, follow-on milk.'* It shows a beautiful, slender ballet dancer beside a cute toddler attempting a pirouette... aaah... how sweet. After this puff of gorgeousness comes the 'science':

Why choose Aptamil with Pronutra Plus Follow-On Milk.
- *Contains 'Omega 3 LCPs'*
- *Enriched with vitamins A C D and Iron*
- *Nutritionally tailored to complement a weaning diet.*

What is Pronutra? Do you know? Does your doctor, midwife or health visitor? Could they tell you where it comes from and its effect on your baby? If it's a 'probiotic', are they aware that 'friendly bacteria' were originally sourced from human faeces? Does the advert tell you that feeds made with water at the correct temperature (70°C) for making up an artificial feed as safely as possible will destroy these 'friendly bacteria'? The companies do not put this fact on their labels, and many even advise using cooler water than is safe to protect the 'friendly bacteria', even though there is no evidence that these darlings make a difference to a baby's health. Vitamins A, C and D and iron sound familiar, but what about vitamin B? Have they left this out? Is it no longer needed? And what about Omega 3 LCPs? Does this mean other milks don't have them? And if it's 'nutritionally tailored' to complement a weaning diet, does that mean that breastmilk or regular infant formula is not? Why would you change from either of these?

What's on the label?
The international body known as Codex* sets the global standards for the essential ingredients in all infant

---

* The Codex Alimentarius Commission (CAC) is the UN food regulatory body which sets the standards for food safety.

formulas and follow-on formulas.* These ingredients should be proven to be essential and do no harm. If a company adds a special 'new' ingredient (not listed in the Codex standards) then this ingredient has not been proved to be essential... or safe. The company is experimenting on your baby.

There is a long, documented list of harm done to infants through contamination, negligence and lack... or excess... of ingredients in the milks. For example, some companies changed the recipe to fit fashionable and unproven nutrition theories.** Babies have suffered or even died, including those born to well-educated parents with excellent living standards. Yet no company has printed on its label: '*This product is as yet unproven to be completely safe, thank you for letting us use your baby as a guinea pig.*' They do not tell you on the label that they put excess vitamins in because they deteriorate over time on the shop's shelf: if your tin is new you might be overdosing your baby, and if it's near the sell-by date there might not be enough. Nor do they all routinely provide and promote the full details for making up artificial feeds as safely as possible (see Appendix 2).

Today, when we believe that the milks and the scrutiny have improved, even the official regulators sometimes admit defeat. Scientists were asked to

---

* I'm using these terms here because that is what Codex uses.

** In 1979 Syntex removed sodium chloride from its infant formula, damaging hundreds of infants. See *The Politics of Breastfeeding*, pp247–249

review the safety of additives used in infant formulas.[*] These experts concluded that, *'few additives have been investigated in relation to their effects on very young children. It is therefore prudent that foods intended for infants under 12 weeks should contain no additives at all.'* [1] In other words, all infant milks for babies under 12 weeks should be made up from fresh ingredients every day and not stored.[**] Codex decided it was not practical to implement this ruling. There was no hue and cry and not a single company put the facts on its labels or in information for health professionals.

Controlled experimentation on tiny babies is rightly judged to be unethical, but this does not stop uncontrolled and invisible experimentation going on all the time as products are 'tested on the market'. Only when many babies, fed on the same product, keep getting a similar serious illness, do problems come to light; sometimes only parental pressure pushes investigation. Do you know any doctor who has sent a tin of milk for laboratory analysis when she or he was diagnosing a sick baby?

But they do promote breastfeeding
But let me get back to the Aptamil advert, which politely asks me to click for more information. It tells me that *'Breastfeeding is Best for Babies'*. Why on earth are they mentioning breastfeeding, when follow-on

---

[*] I use this term because that was the term used in the brief for the scientific committee.

[**] Years ago home-prepared substitutes for breastmilk were made daily from fresh cows' milk, sugar and water.

milks are declared by companies *not* to be substitutes for breastmilk? The advert gives some facts about breastfeeding, including that mixed feeding in the first weeks may reduce breastmilk supply and that I should consider the financial implications of using an infant milk. So far so good, but seeded within this text is a lie that guarantees anxiety and doubt: *'It is important that, in preparation for and during breastfeeding, you eat a healthy, balanced diet.'*

This subtle message cleverly echoes a common belief disproved decades ago. As I mentioned in Chapter 2, lactation is one of the body's most efficient, robust and energy-sparing processes. Women across the world 'fail' to breastfeed for a host of reasons, most notably the baby's access to and behaviour at the breast and the destruction of confidence, but 'a healthy balanced diet' has nothing to do with it.

So why would a company, with access to all the best research, state the opposite?

Breastmilk is used as 'the gold standard', so just mentioning it makes any product sound great. Back in the 1980s, Norwegian sardines were promoted as 'the healthiest food after breastmilk'. This was excellent for sales, but these adverts never implied that sardines were a substitute for breastmilk. The Aptamil advert does. The aim of the marketeer is to make you associate the product with that marvellous stuff, breastmilk, and at the same time plant the idea that breastfeeding is difficult and inadequate. This undermines confidence and creates anxiety.

What's in a name?

It's worth remembering that the infant milk companies were part of the Code's creation. When it was adopted in 1981 they agreed to adhere to it. A cornerstone of the Code is *no public advertising of any substitutes for breastmilk.** So the companies devised a cunning plan. They invented a new product to deliberately evade the Code.

The companies launched 'follow-on milks (FOMs)', claiming that these products were not substitutes for breastmilk, but a replacement for fresh cows' milk. Less modified than regular infant milks, FOMs were cheaper to produce and therefore more profitable. Problems arose when FOMs were launched at a lower price than existing regular infant milks. Their very cheapness tempted poor mothers to feed FOMs to their very young babies, risking hypernatraemia,** which could be fatal.

Now for the clever bit. The design, colour and typeface matched regular infant milk packaging, and made it easy to miss the numbers 1 or 2 after the brand name. And that was the whole point. You were supposed to confuse the two. Brand extention is a powerful tactic used to build an association between

---

* WHO and UNICEF define anything fed to a baby before six months… *'whether suitable or not'*… as a breastmilk substitute. After that, anything that replaces the breastmilk component of the diet for two years or beyond is a breastmilk substitute. These definitions came too late to stop the companies devising their cunning plan.

** Hypernatraemia is a condition when sodium levels in the blood are dangerously high. This can be triggered in infants by the high mineral content of unmodified cows' milk.

product ranges. FOM obliquely advertises infant milk. This cunning plan has worked.

Concerned health authorities and campaigners pressured the companies to equalise the price of both products and change the labels of FOMs. They needed to state they were only suitable from six months of age instead of four months. These moves were essential to protect infants under six months.

Promotion of FOMs chopped and changed claims according to nutritional fashions. FOMs were claimed to prevent iron deficiency anaemia, but research showed they did not. Then they introduced the concept of 'moving on' from breastfeeding, as though you had to stop at six months whether you wanted to or not.

Nutrition experts agreed that babies who were not breastfed should stay on regular infant milk for one year and then change to fresh whole cows' milk as part of a mixed diet.

Once I heard two professors of nutrition roaring with laughter as they agreed that the UK Department of Health's advice to avoid fresh cows' milk until 12 months of age was only because the infant milk companies had lobbied the government. Another truth popped out when a colleague and I attended a launch of a new FOM. When we raised the issue of risk to younger babies, the company representative confessed that their glorious new product was in fact their regular infant milk dressed up as FOM. The company was nervous about harming babies through a spin-off product.

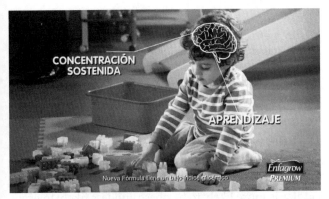

Misleading information in Costa Rica. This ad claims that 'the new formula maintains a low glycaemic index' and that it supports sustained concentration and learning. This is all nonsense.

Unnecessary products

WHO and other health bodies have declared that FOMs are unnecessary products. But no one has managed to stop their production or promotion. Now the companies are pushing 'toddler' and so-called 'growing up' milks, all of which are unnecessary and likely to do harm. For example, because they may contain too much sugar. FOMs are a perfect example of a marketing strategy to sell the same or a similar product tweaked to make you believe that it serves a different purpose.

The importance of impartiality

FOMs are just one example of the insincerity of company promises and the weakness of governments to fulfill theirs. My Aptamil ad was doing exactly what the Code was designed to prevent. It is no worse than other companies' advertising. It pushes an advert at me

> *Persuasion works best when it's invisible. The most effective marketing worms its way into our consciousness, leaving intact the perception that we have reached our opinions and made our choices independently.*
>
> 'The Fake Persuaders', George Monbiot,
> *The Guardian*, 14.05.02

when all I want to do is finish my crossword; it tells lies and withholds information about the risks of artificial feeding. It does not tell me that the cute, pirouetting toddler is more likely to be obese and less likely to grow up to be a slender ballet dancer than if she continues breastfeeding as part of a mixed diet.

To protect all babies, *impartial*, accurate information, without commercial bias, must be available and false information stopped. The Code provides the framework for this essential health measure and it applies universally. Remember the Code is about *marketing*; it is not a health manual. *Some people think the code is a breastfeeding promotion document, but it's not; if 100 per cent of babies were artificially fed, the Code would be even more important.* It is *not* saying you cannot give a baby anything other than breastmilk. It IS saying that companies must not push their products at you, tell lies about infant feeding or withhold vital information. I'm sorry to say most companies still do all three.

The Code was designed to protect *all* babies, regardless of how they are fed. It covers the marketing of *all* substitutes for breastmilk and breastfeeding, including bottles, teats and dummies or any product whose promotion could undermine breastfeeding or the best possible substitute feeding. Most babies are less likely to get ill or die if they're breastfed, so breastfeeding must be protected.

For decades it has been almost impossible to find full and impartial information about artificial feeding products. If a health professional recommended a particular brand, this was rarely based on objective evidence. The UK charity First Steps Nutrition Trust investigates facts about infant feeding products on the UK market and publishes unbiased information about their quality and use. This includes information and marketing to health professionals. Its work is a model of excellence.[2]*

You cannot give advice on artificial feeding unless you have full, impartial information. I am not aware of any government body in any country that provide this. Companies cannot be impartial. As Professor George Kent from the University of Hawaii explains:

> ...standard infant formula and the many variations on it are better than some other methods of feeding and worse than others. On that basis one should not speak of the advantages of breastfeeding, but of the harms associated with other methods of feeding. There is a need to give attention not only to whether infant formula is safe, but also to whether it is effective in doing what it is supposed to do, its functionality. Saying that a food won't make you sick right away is not the same as saying that it meets your needs.[3]

---

* see www.firststepsnutrition.org

A LITTLE ADVICE

Until now I have resisted giving any advice about artificially feeding a baby but I will now. If a baby is not breastfed and under 12 months, a standard infant milk designed for babies under six months is appropriate. If the child is not breastfed and over 12 months, the 'milk' component of the diet should be fresh, plain whole cows' milk (no added sugar). Follow-on, toddler and growing up milks are unnecessary and may make the child less healthy in the long term. They are likely to contribute to overweight and could foster a taste for sweet foods and drinks. This may lead to food preferences associated with type 2 diabetes and heart disease. In some regions of the world, fresh milk from other 'milch' animals may be used.

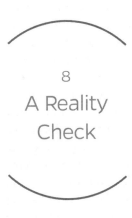

8

A Reality
Check

Experience declares that man is the only animal which devours his own kind, for I can think of no milder term to apply to the general prey of the rich on the poor.

Thomas Jefferson (1743–1826)

This is not history

From time to time I meet people who say: 'Oh yes, the Nestlé boycott. My mum did that, she wouldn't have Néscafe in the house or let me eat their chocolate. They pushed powdered milk onto poor mothers didn't they… and they mixed it with dirty water and the babies died. That was terrible, wasn't it?'

Some people assume that the 'baby food issue' was fixed by the Nestlé boycott. Unethical marketing of baby milk is still happening and it's far more sophisticated than in the era of the 'milk nurses'. It entices and manipulates health professionals and their institutions, politicians and some aid agencies. At best the companies' power and financial influence restrains moral efforts; at worst it shapes policies and action to their advantage. Despite the decades of damage and scandal, companies still invest millions in marketing and promotion of feeding products for babies; this should be zero. Any money spent on disseminating information about their products should not be promotional. It must be directed to health professionals, be scientific and factual only, and with no idealised images or language. As agreed in the Code.

Before we go on, I want to remind you that the majority of people in our world live in conditions where the consequences of not breastfeeding are devastating. Introducing artificial feeding into vulnerable communities, which are not equipped to support it, is immoral. And not just because of dirty water. You sabotage a woman's power and confidence to sustain her baby's health and life. You can destroy a household's economy, depriving an entire family of adequate food and necessities. You make artificial infant feeding aspirational. You create dependency. You increase sickness and death. By accepting the promotion of artificial feeding you become complicit.

To feed a baby artificially as safely as is possible, you need to have access to: a reliable supply of water for hand-washing, sterilisation of equipment and mixing the feed; enough fuel to heat the water to 70°C for every feed; sanitation and waste removal to lessen the risk of infection; literacy and education to read and understand the instructions; and of course enough money to buy the equipment and afford an adequate long-term supply of infant milk.

Let's help put this into context with a quiz* about our world today:

1. How many litres of water do you use every day?
2. How many people live more than a kilometre from a source of water?
3. Are there more people with a toilet or a mobile phone?
4. How many people have access to electricity?
5. How many households have a fridge?
6. What proportion of people can read and write?
7. How many people who need them can access eye tests and glasses?
8. How many people have access to essential health services?
9. How many people live on less than US$4 per day?

The damage that can be done

Vietnam was once a breastfeeding society. However after recovering from the war with the USA (1955–75), rapid economic development attracted the baby food companies to swoop in. Their aggressive marketing and the increased availability of infant milks changed Vietnam into a mixed feeding culture.

Breastfeeding rates plummeted and by 2012 only 17 per cent of babies under six months were exclusively breastfed and just 20 per cent were breastfeeding at all after six months.[1] The companies were spending over US$35 million a year on advertising; 98 per cent of this

---

* Answers at the end of the chapter.

on TV adverts costing US$3,000 for 30 seconds at peak time. The likes of Danone, Abbott, Nestlé, Mead Johnson and others were investing US$24 for every Vietnamese baby born. The 1 in 5 children with stunted growth were testament to their effectiveness.

Not only does this marketing damage health, but it also undermines economic progress. When you consider a 1.5kg tin of Danone's Dumex infant milk costs the equivalent of US$26, and the average factory worker in Vietnam earns under US$7 a day,[2] you realise they would need to work for four days to afford one tin of infant milk. Inequality rises as national income booms. Vietnam has reduced poverty, but many families still struggle. The hard-working Vietnamese are now wasting a modest rise in income on unnecessary products that replace breastmilk and the healthy and delicious solid foods of the traditional Vietnamese diet.

Parents are not stupid, but when, for example, a tin of Mead Johnson's Enfalac A+ claims to be 'clinically proven to support brain development', how do they know this is a lie? Surely no government would allow that? Nutritionist Roger Mathisen, who works in Vietnam, says that people see advertising as a source of facts. The companies know this and tailor their promotion to maintain the illusion.

After counting the human and financial costs of inadequate breastfeeding, Vietnam is now changing. If they revive optimal breastfeeding practices, they will save 2,011 children's lives each year and the anguish of parents coping with the misery of a sick baby. They will also prevent 473 annual deaths from breast cancer. They will save US$23 million a year on treating childhood infections.[3]

The Vietnamese government has recently adopted the Code, with the intention of providing six months state funded maternity leave and breastfeeding support at work. Although this will cost around US$30 million a year, the return on investment will mean that they more than double their money.* Intelligence will rise, health costs go down and lives will be saved.

Who's in charge?

Much of the money needed for this investment is initially coming from the Bill and Melinda Gates Foundation. If the Vietnamese government had been able to honour its commitment to the Code by banning promotion and providing objective information, this private money would not be needed. I do not have space to go into the pros and cons of philanthropy, but this situation raises concerns about buying power and influence, however well-intentioned the outcome. Who should pay for the damage inflicted on infant feeding? Who decides which country gets help? Who should make the necessary changes? Are the wrongdoers ever accountable? Is there a legal process? What precedent does this set? Who is ultimately in control? We all need to consider these matters.

Perhaps we should say that we must forgive and forget and let bygones be bygones, but globally there are no bygones. The shamelessness of the continued marketing is astonishing. Market analyst Euromonitor noted:

In many developing markets, with the notable

---

* US$2.39 for every US$1 invested.

exception of India*, formula advertising can use celebrity endorsement and make claims (such as stating that their products have the same nutritional content as breast milk) that are no longer permitted in most developed markets.[4]

So the advice from the marketing experts is, if your government doesn't give a damn or is under their thumb, infant milk companies can feel free to broadcast falsehoods.

Most of the big infant milk companies claim to respect the Code. At its 2016 AGM Nestlé's CEO Peter Brabeck repeated his usual statement that, 'We must not forget that it was at Nestlé's recommendation that the WHO Code was created, and that ever since the Code was established Nestlé has respected it.' **

Part of the art of marketing is to repeat a lie so often that it becomes perceived as truth.

A case in point

In Turkey in 2013, Danone launched a promotion campaign for their FOM Aptamil 2*** that warned mothers that they could not produce enough breastmilk to meet their babies' needs after six months. The company suggested mothers use FOM to make up the shortfall. Another lie. This deceitful marketing message

---

* India has adopted the Code as a law.

** Translated from the French: *'Parce qu'il ne faut pas oublier que c'etait la recommandation de Nestlé de créer le code de WHO et que des le code il était etabli, Nestlé s'engage de le respecter.'*

***The same product distracting me from my crossword in chapter 7.

> *Endorsement by association, manipulation by assistance.*
> Dr Derrick Jelliffe's description of the relationship between health professionals and the milk companies

boosted infant milk sales in Turkey by 15 per cent. Any woman breastfeeding at six months can continue for as long as she and her baby want to. If a mother had wanted to stop breastfeeding she should have used a standard infant milk, not a FOM.

To its everlasting shame, the Turkish National Paediatric Society endorsed Danone and backed the campaign. We have to ask how Turkish paediatricians were induced to ignore scientific evidence and risk the wellbeing of children and their mothers?

The happy marriage between health professionals and the infant food companies evidently continues to blossom.

Answers to quiz on page 77:
1. This depends on where you live: UK 150 litres; Australia 500 litres; USA over 570 litres; Bangladesh 46 litres; Mozambique 4 litres. Flushing a toilet uses about 15 to 26 litres a day. The essential hygiene (boiling water, frequent hand washing, sterilising all equipment) for artificial feeding is impossible if you don't have a water tap in your home. In low and middle-income countries (poorest and poor) a third of all health facilities lack a safe water source. Water-related diseases affect more than 1.5 billion people every year.
2. Just over a billion (one in seven) people live more than a kilometre away from a water source. Women and children are the water carriers and commonly carry 20 litres (20kg) on their heads over an average 3.7 miles (in Africa and Asia), sometimes spending up to six hours a day.

3. More people have a mobile phone (7 billion) than a toilet: 2.3 billion people lack sanitation. Out of the 2.7 million population of Ekiti state in Nigeria, 1.8 million must defecate wherever they can find a corner. In Dhaka, Bangladesh (Greater Dhaka population 17 million) in one area 40 houses (200 people) share one toilet. Dhaka has just one sewage treatment centre and 80% of solid waste is dumped in open drains. London, UK (population 8.6 million) has 350 sewage treatment centres. Globally a third of all schools lack toilets or any access to safe water and sanitation. For this reason, girls miss school when they're menstruating.

4. 1.2 billion people have no access to electricity. Three billion people cook on open fires or stoves burning wood, animal dung, crop waste or coal. The inhaled pollution causes 4 million early deaths a year, including children under five. The extra fuel needed to make up infant feeds can use up to half the household income while increasing lethal pollution.

5. Globally there are 1.4 billion domestic fridges or freezers and over 7 billion people, but the richer countries have most. In Peru just 45% of households own a fridge; in India it is 27%.

6. One in five people cannot read or write and more of them are women. In Pakistan the male and female literacy rates are 69% and 45%, so most men can read and most women cannot. Literacy is essential for artificial feeding. The label instructions are vital. Often illiterate grandmothers or servants are responsible for artificially feeding the baby.

7. One in ten people with some visual impairment have no access to eye tests or eyeglasses. So even when someone is literate, if they cannot see the words or pictograms on a label, they cannot make up a feed as safely as is possible.

8. 400 million people cannot access essential health services. Across 37 countries, 17% of the population are tipped into poverty (US$2/day) when they must pay for basic treatment. Any artificially fed child is at higher risk of illness. A rich family can pay for treatment, a poor family can be broken by such an event.

9. More than 3.5 billion people, about half of humanity, live on $4 per day or less.

Sources: BBC Radio 4: A Dirty Little Secret 2.4.16, *Doing Good Better* by William Macaskill, FAO, *The Economist*, UNESCO, UNICEF, Vision Aid Overseas, Water Aid, WHO, 2016.

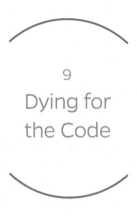

9

Dying for
the Code

*It should not be the corporate greed that feeds
the future, it should be the mothers*

Ines Fernandez[*]

Who runs your country?

The health experts and campaigners who had worked
to get the Code adopted banded together, calling
themselves 'The International Baby Food Action
Network', or IBFAN. Were they unrealistic to believe that
the Code could stop unethical marketing? I don't think
so. Government leaders are shamed by infant death
rates and sick children do no good to their nations. At
every World Health Assembly where infant feeding is
discussed, ministers of health or their delegates make
fine speeches about their commitment to making the

---

* Ines Fernadez of IBFAN, The Philippines, speaking in the film
Milk by Noemi Weiss.

Code work. IBFAN's purpose has been to help them.

We can look back over the past 35 years and see that governments have implemented the Code with varying degrees of commitment and effectiveness. Brazil is a good example. Nestlé had established its market early in the 20th century, and by the 1970s Brazilian mothers breastfed on average for around two months. Infant disease was rife and death rates were high. Over several decades, Brazil's wide-ranging and creative national programmes reversed the decline of breastfeeding. The regulation of marketing was a key part of its strategy. The Brazilian Code was one of the most intelligently drafted in the world and better implemented than in most countries. By 2006, Brazilian mothers' were breastfeeding for an average of 14 months. In 21 years the infant death rate fell by 67 per cent.[1]

Another impressive feat was the initiative of one small, poor country suffering bloody civil war and entrenched poverty: Guatemala. The Guatemalan government implemented the Code effectively and it really worked. The decline in breastfeeding was reversed, reducing infection, malnutrition and deaths. A system of warnings, fines and prosecutions burst the bubble of baby food marketing. Then US company Gerber refused to remove baby pictures from its labels, illegal under the Code. Legal action started. Gerber got the US government to threaten cancellation of a vital trade treaty, an act that would have destroyed the fragile Guatemalan economy. The judge eventually ruled in Gerber's favour. Other poor countries grew wary.

The Philippines

What about larger countries with complex problems, or 'challenges' as the UN documents coyly call them? One example is the Philippines, a former US colony that never shook off its old master's hold. Global corporations held more real power than the government. Infant feeding giants included Abbott, Fonterra, Mead Johnson, Nestlé and Wyeth. A culture of corruption, a low-wage economy and a growing population,* combined with a relatively high literacy rate, made the Philippines an attractive prospect. Millions lived in slums, including about half of the capital Manila's citizens. Thousands lived by scavenging waste. The infamous 'Smokey Mountain', a two million tonne rubbish dump on the edge of Manila, was home and workplace to 30,000 people; the conditions made artificial feeding potentially lethal.

Back in the 1970s, before the Code existed, Filipina paediatrician Dr Natividad Clavano (1932–2007) had torn down the milk company posters, locked up the free samples and asked the salesmen to leave her hospital. She spoke for many when she declared, '*We allowed the companies to touch the lives of our babies, not because we did not care, but because we did not realize the consequences of granting such a privilege.*'[2]

Years later, Filipino health professionals could not claim ignorance of the consequences of allowing companies free reign. They now knew that artificial feeding played a key part in infant illness and death.

---

* In 2006 the population was 87 million and by 2014 it had increased to 100 million.

They witnessed the saggy skins of dehydrated babies, the nappies and sheets soiled with diarrhoea, the rasping, rapid breathing of infant pneumonia. They recorded the deaths. They heard the mothers crying.

The government of the Philippines had voted an enthusiastic yes to the Code in 1981. The minister of health knew that a functioning Code would improve health and save lives. It was essential to transform hospital practices, keep mothers and babies together, stop routine bottle feeds after birth and ban free samples and supplies. You might think that politely telling companies that you had no need of their 'charity' would be easy and save them a lot of money and bother. On the contrary; the companies resisted fiercely and cited the Code's permission. One clause, drafted with orphanages in mind, allowed donations of infant milk to institutions. Company lawyers now claimed that hospitals counted as institutions. Never mind the legal details, ask yourself why a company would fight to give stuff away?

When a gift is not a gift

Free supplies were, and are, a dream marketing tactic, so much so that companies have paid (bribed?) hospitals thousands of dollars to accept them, often with government connivance. Companies know that free supplies sabotage breastfeeding. When more than enough artificial milk to feed every single newborn is dumped in a maternity ward, it gets used. Confronted with a weeping mother and a screaming baby, it's easier for an overworked (and inadequately trained in breastfeeding support) nurse, doctor or midwife to hand out a bottle than sort out the difficulty. Supplies get used as free samples. When a mother goes home with a 'gift' of a tin of artificial milk, 'just in case', her confidence is being undermined.

In those first few days, a moment of doubt can make a mother turn to that tin of milk. Research shows that mothers stick to the brand given in the hospital. Within a few weeks, a mother is a captive customer. If that mother really did want to artificially feed, she has had no full, impartial information and she's been tricked into using a brand that appears medically endorsed. This is not a safe or informed way to embark on artificial feeding.

Samples are used as supplies and supplies are used as samples. They are both banned because they do so much harm. The rule is that if infant milk is needed, the donor must guarantee a continued supply for as long as the baby needs it, perhaps a year or more. This ruling is vital in disasters and emergencies, where haphazard and unsupervised infant milk donations worsen an already dangerous situation for the survival of children.

Back to the Philippines

There was an active IBFAN group, committed staff in the Department of Health (DOH), and health professionals who wanted the Code implemented. But a growing population with a high birth rate was just too juicy a bait for the companies. They were determined to scupper the Code. Because of their influence over the government, the companies were included in the Code drafting process. No surprise then, when public adverts were allowed if vetted by a committee.

In 1992, the launch of UNICEF's Baby Friendly Hospital Initiative motivated the government to introduce a Breastfeeding and Rooming-In Law. Astonishing to think you even needed a law to stop mothers and babies being separated at birth, but the industry wasn't having it. Its representative body* challenged the law claiming that rooming-in was dangerous and increased infection. Through skilled evidence-gathering by DOH doctors, the law went through.

By 2002, the Philippines had established Baby Friendly practices in 1,047 hospitals and a flourishing system of breastfeeding support. Infant death rates were falling, but the committee that vetted adverts was by now the companies' tool. TV adverts for infant milks from birth (banned in most countries) showed beautiful mothers bottle-feeding contented babies to a background of romantic music. As the music faded, a monotone voice gabbled the 'breastfeeding is best' mantra, sending a message that the product was equivalent to breastmilk, the very thing the Code was designed to stop. In that same year, a new international initiative – the 'WHO/UNICEF Global Strategy for Infant and Young Child Feeding'[3] – emphasised implementation of the Code *as a matter of urgency.*

By 2007, the movers and shakers were exhausted, political will had faded and the companies had scaled up

---

* Infant and Paediatric Nutrition Association of the Philippines (IPNAP).

their marketing tactics. The film *Formula for Disaster*[4] shows parents reciting how an infant milk brand makes a baby more intelligent. A salesperson explains how she provides doctors with travel and accommodation for conferences, and extra gifts. All illegal acts. The companies were spending US$100 million a year on advertising, confident that few politicians would dare challenge them. The slums were still there, a third of the population lived on less than US$1 a day and a tin of infant milk cost about US$6.

The Philippines' DOH issued implementation rules for the Code. The Philippines baby food representative body filed a restraining order in the Philippines Supreme Court. The judge rejected their case, stating: *'The framers of the constitution were well aware that trade must be subjected to some form of regulation for the public good. Public interest must be upheld over business interests.'* Both WHO and UNICEF publicly welcomed this decision.

Then Thomas Donahue, President of the US Chamber of Commerce,* wrote to the Philippines' president Gloria Arroyo warning her of *'the risk to the reputation of the Philippines as a stable and viable destination for investment'* if she did not *'re-examine the regulatory decision'.* Four days later the Supreme Court reversed its decision. The separation of legislature and government are enshrined in the constitutions of both the USA and the Philippines.

Public protest came from within and outside the country, together with support from the WHO and UNICEF representatives, who were duty-bound

---

* Still president of the USCC as I write in 2016.

to support implementation of the Code. Suddenly the representatives of both WHO and UNICEF were 'promoted' to positions in other countries. The Philippines' Department of Health requested senior government lawyer Nestor J. Ballocillo to contest the Supreme Court's decision. Soon after, both Nestor and his 21-year-old son were shot dead in the street near their home. No one has ever been charged with these murders.

Observing these struggles for most of my life, what strikes me is that this is not a clash between saints and devils. It is a conflict of purpose betwen the interests of the public good and the interests of companies' profits. Do we want unelected companies to control the decisions, policies, and actions of our elected governments and the UN?

What impresses me is the courage of individuals who risk so much, even their lives, to do the right thing.

Here is an account of one Nestlé employee who suffered for behaving morally.

The salesman's story

In 1994, Syed Aamir Raza was thrilled when, aged 24, he got a job as a salesman with Nestlé Pakistan. His job was to promote infant food products and increase sales. He was given a brand new motorbike to do his rounds. He had never heard of the Code and was not told about it in his training. He was instructed to say 'breast is best' quickly before his sales pitch, to give free Cerelac* samples to mothers and to talk about the range of infant milks.

---

* Cerelac is a cereal-based complementary food for babies.

He had an allowance for gifts for health professionals such as air tickets or perfume. Some doctors asked for more. When one demanded an air conditioner, Aamir asked his line manager, who said, 'OK, but Nan and AL100* sales should go up.' In 1996, Nestlé created its 'Charter', its own rather fuzzy version of the Code, and Aamir received his personal copy.** He read it and was astonished. The 'Charter' stated that Nestlé did not give gifts to doctors, contact mothers or use sales incentive schemes.

A few months later Aamir was waiting to speak to a paediatrician, Dr Diamond Emmanuel. They had become friends, despite the fact that he refused all gifts. Diamond arrived looking serious; he had come straight from the painful task of telling a mother and father that their baby had just died. 'Why did the child die?' Aamir asked. 'Because of people like you,' replied Diamond. Aamir was stunned and as he left the office he saw and heard the grieving parents.

Despite having a wife and children to support, Aamir resigned from his job and returned the motorbike. He kept copies of all the documents that proved the truth of the sales practices. His next step was one of great courage and great innocence. With his father's help, he wrote a 'Legal Notice' and sent 80 pages of damning evidence to Nestlé Pakistan, asking it to 'withdraw all its infant products from the Pakistan market' and 'to terminate service of staff involved in non-professional

---

* Brand names of Nestlé baby milks.

** Nestlé published this 'Charter' as part of its campaign to persuade the Church of England to drop its boycott.

and unethical practices within 15 days.'

Every time I read these words I want to cry. It reminds me of a gazelle trotting over to drink from a pool where the crocodiles are waiting. Many modern Davids slink away from modern Goliaths, but Aamir was a true David.

Aamir informed WHO Pakistan of the violations against the Code. They told him they could do nothing as their role was merely advisory. Then WHO did something disgraceful. Without his permission, it passed his letter to the District Health Officer and Nestlé soon had access to it. By this time Aamir had contributed to the evidence-gathering of the IBFAN group in Pakistan, who had witness statements describing Nestlé and other companies' flouting of the Code. Life became really difficult for all involved. Shots were fired at Aamir's house and he received death threats. His family moved out of town and he fled the country. He became a refugee and was separated from his family for seven years. His parents died and he could not even return for their funerals. Eventually his wife and children were able to join him.

In 2014, a version of Aamir's story was told in the film *Tigers* by Oscar-winning director Danis Tanovich. I recommend it.

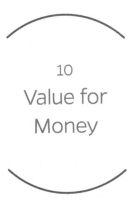

10
Value for
Money

*Equality for women demands a change in the
human psyche... It means valuing parenthood
as much as we value banking.*

Polly Toynbee

Who does the work?

Women have always been economically active. For most
of human existence they have been the main providers
of food... the breadwinners.* No gatherer/hunter
(most humans who have ever lived) or farmer would
have stopped breastfeeding because she was working.
Breastfeeding was as important as gathering fruits,

---

* Researchers have deduced that in most human groups women
gathered or foraged a range of foods and caught small animals,
contributing far more in terms of daily nutrients than the 'big game'
hunts that mostly men undertook. When agriculture evolved, women
did the bulk of the labour, as they still do today in much of the world.

leaves, small animals or seafood or harvesting grains and roots. Until industrialisation transformed our lives, there was little division between work and home, between earning a living and 'domestic' life; dovetailing these tasks was skillfully managed.

Division of labour according to sex has varied throughout time and between societies, castes and classes. An 18th century observer of rural English life wrote, '*In the long winter evenings, the husband cobbles shoes, mends the family clothes and attends to the children while the wife spins.*'[1] A century later, both men and women worked long hours at machines in noisy, dangerous factories, unable to attend to their children. They had no choice; rural production had been eclipsed. The spinner at home could pause to feed her baby, but she could not stop an industrial machine or defy the factory master. Whether in or out of the home, industrialisation increased women's work burdens and they lost control of the interweaving of childcare and work.

Despite this, the 1881 British Census excluded women's household tasks from the category of productive work. Until then economic activity had been recorded at 98 per cent for women. After 1881, only 42 per cent of women were officially recorded as contributing to the economy. In the 21st century, in both rich and poor societies, there is still a big bias and a muddle about women's economic contribution.

Who is the economy for?
When a mother buys infant milk and bottles, money

goes from her pocket into the manufacturer's. Even the artificial milk industry acknowledges the superiority of breastmilk and its delivery method, so why are its producers poorer than the makers of the inferior product? Carolyn Campbell has summarised the denial of the economic value of breastmilk:

> *The discussion of whether or not breastmilk is the ideal infant food is like asking whether or not the kidneys are the ideal means to eliminate wastes from the body and suggesting that dialysis machines ought to replace human kidneys. Human breastmilk is controversial because it is a highly valued product produced by the family for family consumption, and at least up to now has been totally removed from capitalist market control. Subsistence production is contrary to the needs of capital which, to be effective, must incorporate into the market as many goods necessary for or 'desired' by humans. Without commodity production and distribution via the market, there is no surplus value extraction, i.e. no profit.*[2]

People have tried to commoditise and profit from donated breastmilk. They miss the point. Breastfeeding is far more than transfer of breastmilk. It is a relationship between two people.

Economic structures are supposed to make human life better. Currently we live in a world where humans exist to serve what is called 'the economy', but the economy does not serve most humans. By the end of

2009, US$14 trillion of Western governments' money was used to bail out failing banks.[3] By the end of 2011, at least US$5 billion of this taxpayers' money was directly used to pay the million dollar bonus of 5,000 individual traders and bankers.[4] Two and a half billion people don't even have a bank account.[5] Our global system values making money for money's sake. Breastfeeding is a capital investment. Where are women's bonuses?

Natural capital

Back in the 1970s the World Food Conference rejected Norway's proposal to include human milk in world food production statistics. I have not found out why, but perhaps the scientists used to dealing with rice yields and numbers of tractors simply could not cope with something so… female? Almost 50 years later a key review[6] of global food production gave the powerful message that 30 to 50 per cent (1 to 2 billion tonnes) of all food produced on this planet is lost before it reaches the human stomach. Breastmilk is never mentioned, although its universal suppression is part of this wastage.

Withdraw breastfeeding and whole societies would collapse. One study showed that in eight West African countries, mothers contributed an estimated one billion litres of human milk annually to their nations' food supplies. Replacement with artificial feeding would cost an annual US$412 per infant that's more than US$1 a day in a region where most families live on less than US$1 a day.[7] The resulting health costs would drain all public funds and infant and young child death rates would soar. Here is a primary resource. If the financial gurus persuaded governments (and such persuasion is their business) to provide some form of payment for a mother's public health contribution, that money would recirculate into the general economy.

Cash transfers work. In Ethiopia, the Productive Safety Nets Programme (PSNP) provided 7.2 million people with 30 Birr (US$3.50) per head per month. Mothers spent the money on nutritious local food, soap, children's clothes and healthcare. In general, women use money more wisely than men do. Micro-credit systems, when banks and governments provide small loans for poor women to set up modest income-generating enterprises, have been remarkably successful. Women repay loans more reliably than conventional businessmen.

However, international financial institutions such as the World Bank and the International Monetary Fund (IMF) have bullied countries into policies that blank out and deny much of the economic contribution of women.

In 1997, the World Bank offered a US$20 million loan to Macedonia to reform its primary health care system, on condition that maternity leave be reduced from nine to three months. Thankfully UNICEF pointed out the increased health costs of women stopping breastfeeding early, and the condition was dropped. The WB had not counted women breastfeeding and caring for their own babies as an investment, even if it saved millions in healthcare and social costs.

Governments and commercial companies 'invest'

billions in expensive new technology – roads, bridges, airports, dams or power generation plants – 'for the good of society'. The crucial primary investment in the emotional, physical and mental health of all humans, which breastfeeding and mothering provide, is invisible.

Absurd accounting

New Zealand economist Marilyn Waring was one of the first to challenge the denial of women's contribution to the global economy.[8] The UN System of National Accounts (UNSNA), the established worldwide method of assessing economic 'health', excluded crucial productive activities. Home food production, protection of the environment, caring for children, aged, sick or disabled relatives, home-making, helping neighbours and all the varied tasks that mostly women do, counted for nothing in the UNSNA system. Weapons manufacture, polluting the environment (e.g. carbon trading or building a coal-fired power station) and even the earnings of a pimp counted (national systems include circulating money from the 'hidden economy'). Every officially recorded activity that harms the Earth is seen to benefit the 'health' of the economy, yet caring for a new human is viewed as an expense and not a contribution, unless products are bought.

According to dominant economic doctrines, if the Amazon is entirely 'developed' then Brazil's economy will be the envy of the world. But it will be a world where humans cannot live.

> *Destroying the rainforest for economic gain is like burning a Renaissance painting to cook a meal.*
>
> E. O. Wilson, biologist

Breastfeeding economics

In a money-obsessed world, I'm a bit uncomfortable with the economic evaluation of breastfeeding, but it is a language the powerful understand. As Australian economists Julie Smith and Lindy Ingham explain: *'While some may find putting a price on mothers' milk offensive, putting no price on it suggests that it has no value'.*[9]

In 1993, the UNSNA international accounting guidelines were revised to reflect some unpaid work in households and called the UN System of National Accounting 93 (SNA93). Australia took SNA93 on board. Indeed, one national accountant commented that ignoring unpaid household activities had not been a matter of economic principle, but merely a practical convenience. In other words, it was just too much bother to work it all out. I feel much the same about my tax returns, but punishment awaits me if I don't do them. It seems that government economists are allowed to dump the tricky bits.

Now in Australia the value of home-produced fruit, vegetables, meat, eggs, beer and wine are included in the Gross Domestic Product (GDP). In 1997 all this home production amounted to A$1 billion. Production includes services as well as goods. Australian economists recommended that the value of unpaid service work, such as childcare, domestic chores and voluntary work, should be taken into account.

The way to do this (economists love a complex system, even if it baffles the rest of us) is to pop these values into so-called 'satellite accounts'. These are separate from the core national accounts, which record all the market transactions (commercial sales and services), but are still consistent with them. Now I am not sure I quite understand, but I see it like this: 'We have a clever bank account system, but you are not quite important enough to use it. But we can value the coins in your piggy bank and we will count them regularly and acknowledge they exist.' Of course we know that one motive is to gather taxes, but even then it is a step in the right direction in terms of acknowledging the invisible work people, especially women, do.

But environmental and human capital assets are not yet included in national balance sheets. Something needs to be 'processed' in some way before it can have value. The value of reproductive work – that is, giving birth, breastfeeding and providing the consistent responsiveness that all babies need – is ignored by accountants and economists.

Most studies have calculated the value of breastmilk by comparing it with artificial milk, but that is a poor comparison. It is as though you valued a mahogany forest as equal to a potted plant.

Julie and Lindy explored different methods of valuing breastfeeding in economic terms, but the one I understand best is as an estimate of a nation's capital assets.

Think of a natural resource like oil, gas or a gold mine, a skilled and intelligent workforce or a big telecommunications company. These all make a country rich. These Australian economists calculated the capitalised value of breastfeeding in their own country to be around A$37 billion. This was comparable with the value of the giant Australian telecommunications company Telstra, valued at A$30 billion at the time they published their work. This far exceeded the value of livestock (A$17.9 billion) and plantation forests (A$4.5 billion).

If Australian women were supported to practice optimal breastfeeding, then the value of breastfeeding and human milk production would be A$100 billion. Three times its current level and three times the value of Telstra. The folly of the conventional accounting system was that when breastfeeding declined over the decades, Australia appeared richer. Whenever breastfeeding increases and sales of infant milks and bottles reduce, the accounts show this as a decline in economic output. This is ridiculous.

The latest research[10] into the economic impact of breastfeeding shows that achieving optimal breastfeeding rates would enable people to achieve the potential they were born with; in terms of both health and intelligence. This would enhance natural capital.

Making it count

Family size is related to female education and equality. When women have the opportunity to participate in worthwhile and valued occupations, they take control of their reproductive lives. The aim of the Fifth UN Sustainable Development Goal* is to achieve gender equality and empower all women and girls. This means increased female participation in education, the labour market and politics. Quite right too. What must be addressed is whether women's inclusion in the labour market, without well-planned and financially-supported provision for breastfeeding and mothering, will lead to more separation for babies, less breastfeeding and more exploitation of an underclass of poorly paid child carers.

If breastfeeding and mothering were economically valued and supported, then mothers might feel more confident and less ambivalent about breastfeeding. When Sheila Kitzinger declared that the only reason a woman should not breastfeed was if she did not want to, her vision was of a world where all health workers would be properly trained and the lies of commercial promotion stopped. She saw a future where women could be confident to breastfeed without physical, emotional or economic pain.

---

* The UN Sustainable Development Goals, otherwise known as the Global Goals, are a universal call to action to end poverty, protect the planet and ensure that all people enjoy peace and prosperity. They build on the successes of the Millennium Development Goals, while including new priorities such as climate change, economic inequality, innovation, sustainable consumption, peace and justice.

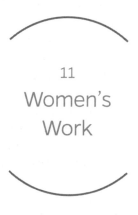

11
Women's Work

How hard a life her servant lives.
W.B. Yeats (1865–1939)

Maria's life does not count

Maria and her husband José live in their earth-floored, two-roomed wooden house in a remote region of Guatemala. Set in a third of a hectare (0.8 acres) of land, it's about five hours' hard walking from the nearest rough road. They have an outside tap with water piped from a spring and a well-maintained latrine. They have brought up eight healthy children (the eldest is 27), all born at home with only José's help, and all breastfed for two or three years. They feed their family entirely from their own labour with maize and beans from the communal cultivation area. Around their house they produce vegetables and fruit, keep chickens and turkeys, a pig, fish in a little pond and two coffee bushes. They gather wild foods such as river snails, and honey from a semi-wild beehive. The local cash crop is cardamom and when world prices go up, so does their cash income. Any money is spent on sugar, soap, candles, clothes and, when possible, their children's education. In monetary value they are very poor, but the family has not gone hungry.

In her forties and illiterate, Maria was chosen by her community to take the government-sponsored training course to become a birth attendant. She has since supported 19 women through birth; exclusive breastfeeding is the norm and problems are unknown. All 19 mothers and babies did well, except for one baby who died at three weeks, after being flown with his mother to the nearest hospital. The only emergency transport is a light aircraft owned by the local 'narco baron'.*

Maria and José are much respected by their community. Maria's skills and knowledge make her one of the most productive women I have ever met, and certainly one with a 'zero-carbon footprint'. Yet her outstanding contribution to society is invisible. Everything she does is not counted. A US citizen owns the land their community cultivates. If he decides to reclaim it for cattle rearing, which economists see as the profitable thing to do, the whole village would need food aid or go hungry. Local water sources would become polluted (cattle cause water contamination and

---

* The narco baron is a wealthy drug trafficker.

disease), and tree clearance for grazing would damage the micro-climate, triggering flooding and landslides. Yet any milk and meat sold will be viewed as economic progress in Guatemala's national accounts.

Maria works hard but she is an unstressed, calm woman. After supper in the candlelit house, she cuddles her six-year-old son (her youngest and last child) until he falls asleep. We converse from time to time, but all is peaceful. During her 20 years of pregnancy and breastfeeding she never needed a cushion, a breast pump, a DVD, a book or a YouTube video. She worked at her daily tasks without any sense that she was doing anything special. Though she does not know it, she is at low risk of breast and ovarian cancer. Her children are polite and intelligent and take part cheerfully in the family duties: shutting up the pig and piglets at night, catching fish in the pond, shelling beans, and making tortillas. Maria and José's lives are hard-working, dignified and a great contribution to the health and ecology of their community and country. Yet these lives do not count. Only their monetary share in cardamom sales (or if José does some paid labour) and the cash they spend on candles, sugar or soap, mean anything to economists. If the economy 'improves', the small local shop will sell more soft drinks and processed foods, which will add to the growing problems of obesity already seen in Guatemala's urban areas.

Meanwhile the local 'narco baron', who lives in a mansion over the mountain, keeps cattle, employs staff and buys furniture and luxuries. His contribution counts.

Women friendly?

Almost every traditional society had some system of respite and support for new mothers. Family and neighbours would take over a woman's duties, feed and care for her while she gave birth and established breastfeeding. Some employers accepted family labour systems, where a relative temporarily replaced a mother when she had a new child. This is still the norm for tea pickers in Bangladesh.

Almost a century ago in 1919, the International Labour Organisation (ILO) created the first international convention on maternity leave and breastfeeding breaks for all women. The ILO, now part of the UN, established minimum standards that apply today. In the 21st century, rights for the formally employed are established in many countries. But this is meaningless for the majority of women who work in casual 'hire and fire' employment. Even if they are aware of their rights they cannot, or dare not, claim them.

Women make up half the world's informal work sector, and up to 90 per cent in some countries. The majority of unpaid workers in family businesses are women. Most street vendors, a third of casual agricultural workers, and 40 per cent of construction workers in India are women. Choice is not an issue; they work for their own and their families' survival. They go unpaid when ill or needed to care for a sick child or relative. Domestic workers, fisherwomen, waitresses, bar girls, sex workers and many more work unrecorded and unprotected by any official bodies or systems. This happens in rich countries too. A 2012 survey in the USA found that two-thirds of nannies, housekeepers and home health aides were immigrants, half of whom were undocumented.[1]

In 2000, an internationally agreed ILO Maternity Protection Convention specifically included all women in 'atypical work'. However, a let-out clause enabled countries and companies to postpone or evade full implementation.* How cynical is that?

When US supermarket chain Walmart profits from the low wages and non-existent or non-implemented maternity rights** of its employees worldwide, do shareholders complain? Six months after a Bangladesh factory fire killed 100 workers making clothes for Walmart, 1,000 people died and 2,500 were injured in the collapse of the eight-storey Rana Plaza Building sweatshop complex. Most victims were women.[2] Did western buyers care that bargain fashion comes at such a price? Much economic growth depends on the low-waged labour of poor women who make the low-priced goods that consumer societies demand. Who protects their rights?

When people talk of 'women friendly' policies they often mean tolerating childbearing and childcare as though men had nothing to do with it. If men took responsibility for all child-related tasks, except

---

* 2000 ILO Maternity Protection Convention (C183).

** In the USA, pregnancy and birth are regarded as a 'disability' in relation to claims for any leave. There are no statutory rights for pregnancy, birth and breastfeeding in relation to employment and any that exist are due to individual company policy.

> In the UK, a mother with two children at nursery needs £40,000 a year to profit from going to work. The average full-time woman worker earns £24,202 a year.
>
> *The Sunday Times*, April 2016

for breastfeeding, then they would be the more disadvantaged sex. The few men who act as primary carers throughout their children's lives are the exception. Any efforts towards equalisation of men's and women's work, status and pay has not resulted in a significant proportion of men taking several years away from work to raise children. Status as well as money has a big effect on these decisions. Giving birth and breastfeeding are low-status activities.

Other people's children

Poor women often care for the children of richer women, at the cost of separation from their own. Inez, from the Philippines, left her two-month-old baby with a relative to work as a nanny in the USA: '*The first two years I felt I was going crazy. You have to believe me when I say it was like I was having intense psychological problems. I would catch myself gazing at nothing, thinking about my child*.' Deprived of closeness with her own baby, a nanny often redirects her maternal love to the baby in her care: '*The only thing you can do is to give all your love to the child. In my absence from my children, the most I could do with my situation was to give all my love to that child*'.[3] One professor has called these workers 'emotional proletarians' who 'produce authentic emotions in exchange for a wage.'[4]

Several governments, including Indonesia, Sri Lanka and the Philippines, encourage female migrant labour to boost their economies. A tenth of the Philippines' population works abroad, supporting half the country's households and leaving nine million children missing a parent. Three-quarters of those workers are women. Marriages crumble and mother-child relationships suffer, but this is all 'good for the economy'. Thus the economic machine punishes children, both those separated from migrant worker mothers and those of privileged women. Children can experience emotional damage when mother substitutes are abruptly changed to fit parental careers or petty disputes.

Jealousy of a nanny's skills can be a problem. Wong Siew Mei, a Malaysian businesswoman who employed an Indonesian nanny, told me her story. On returning from work, she asked for her five-month-old son who was sleeping soundly on his nanny's back. *'She suggested I should wait until my son woke up,'* Siew Mei told me. *'So I sacked her. I didn't like it that my son was getting close to her and perhaps preferring her smell to mine.'*

Who holds the baby?

Much of the 20th and 21st centuries' progress towards equal rights and opportunities for women, particularly their inclusion in the workplace, is dependent on the oppression of other women. The essential tasks still need to be done.

I am not suggesting that mothers should stay at home, though if they are able to and want to, I'm not against it. It would be great if that many had a choice. But given sufficient maternity leave to establish breastfeeding, it is not essential. Women find ways to continue breastfeeding for months and years if they are confident and have information and support. It must be actively endorsed by government policy and employment practice. There must be implementation mechanisms so that women can take it for granted that they can continue breastfeeding if they want to. The idea that breastfeeding must cease 'when women return to work', is boosted by milk company promotional messages and supplemented by general ignorance. It's worth noting that a 1980s four-country study found that most artificial feeding was done by mothers who stayed at home, and women who worked outside the home breastfed for longer.[5]

What is missing is the economic, social and cultural prioritising of a small child's needs, while recognising that a mother is a person in her own right. This requires flexibility, imagination and innovation: all the qualities business gurus claim to love. They exist in some progressive countries and companies, but these are unusual. The Scandinavian system of family-friendly policies is still an exception, even though it has benefited these countries' economies. The USA has the least adequate maternity legislation in the rich world. Many women still feel grateful for, not entitled to, fulfilment of their rights. Even professional women can feel sidelined or belittled when they claim their breastfeeding rights at work.

But most mothers are powerless in their workplaces because most are not protected by the systems. That grieving Filipina mother, Inez, could have brought her two-month-old with her to the USA, cared for two children and carried out domestic tasks in a flexible way, as women do all over the world everyday. Then two people would have suffered less. Would immigration bureaucracy or her employer have permitted this? Can this ever be 'the norm'?

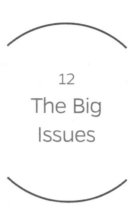

12
The Big
Issues

*Without sufficient public scrutiny, all political
systems degenerate into the service of wealth.*

George Monbiot

Entitlement

In the 1980s the Nobel prize-winning economist,
Amartya Sen, introduced the simple concept that
people do not starve for lack of food, but from lack of
entitlement to food.[1] In the 19th century a million Irish
died of hunger when their potato crops failed, because
they were not entitled to eat the food they produced
for their English landlords. So too with the great
20th century famines in Asia and Africa: people with
money, land, property or connections to the powerful
did not starve to death. Sen's theory has proved robust.
In 1997, the year Ethiopia became a food exporter, I

bought Ethiopian lentils in a British store. Despite the 1980s famines, the World Bank had demanded economic reforms that included the export of grain reserves to repay debt. In 1998 another Ethiopian famine began. The foreign advisers working there maintained their usual bodyweights. You may have noticed that journalists or politicians in famine zones do not faint with hunger before the news cameras. They have entitlement to food.

So too with breastfeeding. There is no shortage of breastmilk or women wanting to breastfeed their babies. If all existing, supportive policies were fully implemented, breastfeeding rates would soar. No other production process is so easy to switch on and off. Women stop breastfeeding because misinformation and inept care crush their confidence and innate skills. Pressures and circumstances beyond their control separate them from their babies. Constraints in health systems; ignorance, commercial lies and greed; inhumane and unimaginative working systems; distorted cultural values and political blindness all come together to destroy the entitlement of women to sustain their children's health and lives, and protect their own bodies.* All over the world there are breastmilk famines; they are not caused by nature but by a loss of entitlement.

Advocate for the right to food George Kent argues that countries that cannot control their own

---

* See The Innocenti Declaration at www.ennonline.net/ iycfinnocentideclaration2005

food systems are susceptible to outside pressures.[2] Breastfeeding is a food system; the country that cannot control the baby food companies' unethical marketing can't protect breastfeeding and all citizens are made vulnerable. Looking at infant feeding in the light, or rather the shadow, of three of the biggest issues facing us and our world in the 21st century, shows just how vulnerable we all are.

Mass migration

We are all the children of migrants. Our ancestors all came out of Africa. Most of us have forebears who fled terror or poverty to save their families or better their lives. Yet today those fleeing war, persecution and economic collapse are rejected and stigmatised by nations supposedly founded on the principles of human decency. No one abandons their home without good reason. In 2016 there are 60 million people (including refugees, asylum seekers, the stateless and returnees) whose lives are a continuum of instability, deprivation and fear; a testament to a shameful lack of humanity among humans. It's estimated that at least 5 million of these displaced people are children under five. They are far more vulnerable to malnutrition and infection than older children and adults.[3]

As this book goes to press the migrant crisis in Europe remains a live crisis. Many of these migrant mothers coming from the Middle East have already had breastfeeding sabotaged. Inept hospital practices and milk marketing existed in Syria, as in many other countries. Mixed feeding and doubts about the robustness of lactation were well established. Many women depended on artificial milks before they fled. As a result, aid workers are faced with huge dilemmas.

Many infants are already artificially fed as they transit and their desperate mothers don't know where their next feed will come from. Aid workers are put in the impossible position of supporting breastfeeding mothers while doing everything they can to protect the non-breastfed infants. Conditions are appalling* and compromises have been huge:** it is a no-win situation. Mistaken beliefs about breastmilk disappearing under stress and a need for supplementation is common. Well-meaning volunteers have distributed untargeted donations of infant milks and feeding bottles. Few know that breastmilk can be re-stimulated and re-established, and frightened, anguished women get angry and distraught. It is an uphill battle against a tide of misinformation and miscommunication.***

The best 'emergency preparedness' is established, resilient breastfeeding practices among empowered mothers. Without this, humanitarian responders are on the back foot, with an ever-present risk to children's health and survival.

---

* Poor water and sanitation, no follow-up, staff shortages, lack of translators and just five minutes' contact time with mothers.

** Infant feeds have been mixed communally in open vats in Greece.

***There are some success stories too – mothers provided with breastfeeding support in mobile safe areas and tents, with 24/7 staff able to react to alerts through social media and respond sensitively with help and information.

Antibiotic resistance

Developed in the 1930s, antibiotics transformed our world, saving millions of lives. Without them we could never have abandoned breastfeeding on the grand scale of the 20th century and still reduced infant and young child deaths.[*] However, antibiotic use in infancy and early childhood is a risk factor for obesity.[4] Their use disrupts our microbiome, the balance of beneficial bacteria in our guts that influences our health and wellbeing.

Antibiotic resistance is global and has reached the drugs of last resort. Lives are being lost that once could be saved. Antibiotics are over-prescribed, sold off prescription and misused worldwide. In many countries they are routinely used as growth promoters for livestock; 90 per cent are excreted in animal urine and excrement and widely dispersed into our environment through fertiliser, groundwater and surface runoff. In the USA, the antibiotics tetracyline and streptomycin are sprayed on fruit trees to act as pesticides.[5]

Of course you know what I'm going to say. If governments invested in the support of women to breastfeed, children would be saved, lifelong immune systems would be improved and health costs would plummet. This could become a matter of life and death for us all when antibiotics become ineffective. Much is already known about this, but investment is low because it is not financially attractive. Governments must take responsibility. The example of blood banks shows that

---

[*] Mass immunisation has also played a major role.

altruism works better than commerce.* Breastmilk banks are never short of donors. Women are eager to give their milk to save the lives of other women's children. When well managed, donation is safer than commerce.[6]

WHO, governments and public health bodies are all worried. In 2016, the UK Chief Medical Officer, Dame Sally Davies, announced that *'Antimicrobial resistance poses a catastrophic threat. If we don't act now, any one of us could go into hospital in 20 years for minor surgery and die because of an ordinary infection that can't be treated by antibiotics. And routine operations like hip replacements or organ transplants could be deadly because of the risk of infection.'*[7]

No one speaks publicly of the inevitable increase in the deaths of babies and small children. It's too ghastly to mention.

Climate change

Climate change is scary. Leading scientists and experts do their best to alert us, but little changes. Wasteful consumption is the driving force of a global economic system that squanders natural resources. Powerful bodies like the World Bank have urged nations to aspire to western values as a driver of this system. It would take three planet Earths for everyone to live like a North American yet financial analysts seem pleased when car sales rise in India and China. News media avoid the latest figures on environmental destruction while they report share prices *ad nauseam*.

---

* See *The Gift Relationship* by Richard Titmuss (LSE Books, 1997).

It's been known for years that the production of cows' milk and red meat puts these products among the most environmentally damaging foods. The two are connected because many beef products come from dead dairy cows and their unwanted male calves.

There is a big difference in environmental costs between the production of ordinary dairy products (fresh milk, cheese, butter) and all the artificial milks.* Greenhouse gas emissions attributable to milk powder are significantly higher because of the additional processing and energy used during manufacture. On average, for every kilo of milk powder produced, four kilos of greenhouse gases are emitted.

Let's look at China and India. China adopted the Code but ignores it, whereas India has brought in effective laws. Both countries have similar population size (around one billion) and both aggressively pursue economic growth.

In the four years up to 2012 China's market for all types of artificial milks for infants and young children grew by 90 per cent. India's market grew by 13 per cent. China emitted 80 times more greenhouse gases (from artificial milks) than India. Market analysts predict continuing sales growth in China. Within nine years (2008 to 2017) China will have increased its greenhouse gas output (from artificial milks) from 1.2 million tonnes to 4.2 million tonnes. That's an increase of 250 per cent.[8]

Are Chinese children better nourished? By the 1990s, China had already established adequate health services

---

* Standard infant formula, follow-on milks, toddler milks, growing-up milks and other silly names.

for all and infant and young child death rates were falling steadily. Breastfeeding was promoted and supported with workplace facilities. They adopted the Baby Friendly Hospital Initiative with enthusiasm and strong government endorsement. Complementary feeding traditions were among the best in the world. But policy changes allowed the big foreign companies to invade. Marketing has duped the Chinese into abandoning their healthy child feeding practices. The result is full participation in the child obesity pandemic with a future of increasing type 2 diabetes and heart disease.

What is to be done?

We must broaden the minds of our politicians before they destroy democracy by handing over all power to the giant transnationals. Already companies take aggressive action against governments' public health decisions. For example, tobacco companies legally challenged the Australian government when it proposed plain packaging for cigarettes. Australia is a rich country with the means and skills to fight off this challenge and they won, for now, but many countries cannot and dare not*. Trade partnerships are being designed to put profits before people's health.[9]

If we are to save our children and our planet we must invest right now. Breastfeeding can provide a significant contribution to combat the major problems of our time. It is 'natural capital' and those who hold

---

* Remember what happened in the Philippines when they tried to resist corporate power through the most conventional and respected of means: the law.

it should be acknowledged and rewarded for sharing it. Governments always find money for an issue they judge to be important, like a war – or in my own country's case – a royal wedding or the costly personal security of former prime ministers. I note that there are many who want to see change so that the purpose of daily life is not the making of money as an end in itself, but the thriving of all people. I see that economics has become a religion. Its dogmas are expressed in a language that few understand. Some (certainly not all) economists and politicians announce that millions must accept deprivation and injustice 'for the good of the economy'.

What good have their edicts done? Since I first wrote about this subject 30 years ago, inequality has stretched beyond all imaginings. Extremes of wealth and deprivation around the world have become obscene. This is not just bad for the poor, but bad for the rich too. There is a direct relationship between social ills and inequality, independent of overall national wealth. The more unequal a society the worse its infant and young child mortality, its rates of obesity, cancer, and heart disease, mental illness, violence and homicide and life expectancy.[10] As I showed in Chapter 1, breastfeeding is the great equaliser: it gives a baby born into poverty a chance to be as healthy and intelligent as one born into wealth.

The great god of the dominant economic doctrine is 'growth'. This may be needed in the poorest nations, but it is unnecessary and even harmful in the richest. 'Growth' is an apt word because it is also used for a tumour that can ultimately destroy the body. The source of thousands of

> *We have to stop leaving all the decision making to the so-called decision-makers, but take matters into our own hands, realise that each of us makes a difference, and that if everyone who cares acts in a way that is ethical... then the world would be changed very fast.*
>
> Jane Goodall

beneficial products, the forests, are destroyed to produce palm oil, soya or other foods that enter our systems of over production, waste and damaging diets. The sea and land are polluted with chemicals that destroy the cycle of life; all this to feed 'growth' because it is 'good for the economy'. Women are led to believe that breastfeeding is not possible, or that it demeans their status or is a trivial pastime, while excess production of cattle colonises poor people's land to end up as products that damage health. The tumour must be fed.

The fact that children get ill and die because of the continued unethical marketing of artificial milks is unacceptable when we know so much about the risks. Every day, governments who have repeatedly promised to resolve this problem are pressured to turn a blind eye and remain complicit. The Convention on the Rights of the Child states that all segments of society have the right to knowledge of breastfeeding.[11] When this knowledge is drowned in a constant stream of commercial untruths, blandishments and bribery, this right is destroyed. This is what is ghastly.

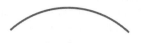

Acknowledgements

I warmly thank my friend and colleague Yasmin Hosny. Her focus, dedication and research and organisational skills have provided a major contribution to this book. It could not have been completed without her.

My editor Zoë Blanc and publisher Martin Wagner have been patient and understanding beyond the call of duty. Maria Pinter's warm and calm welcome is a ray of sunshine. Any author is fortunate to work with these people. I would also like to thank Susan Last, editor of the entire *Why It Matters* series.

I also feel immense gratitude to the following experts and thinkers who have provided information, read drafts, checked facts and talked through problems without complaint: Sue Ashmore, Carol Bartel, Mike Brady, Ian Bray, Janet Calvert, Elsie Chee, David Clark, Alan Dangour, Jan Cornfoot, Helen Crawley,

Diamond Emmanuel, Tom Hale, Elizabeth Hormann, Siobhan Hourigan, Julie Kavanagh, Joo Kean, Sandra Lang, Lida Lhotska, Marie McGrath, Roger Mathisen, Judith Richter, Patti Rundall, Felicity Savage, Vilneide Serva, Mary Smale, Terry Wefwafwa, Noemi Weiss, Zhang Shuyi.

My writers' group colleagues Amy Corzine, Rosemary Hayes, Penny Speller, Victor Watson and Jane Wilson have been most tolerant. I joined them half way through writing a novel when I got waylaid into this venture. Their suggestions and support have been invaluable.

I thank my husband John, my children Frances and Nathaniel and their partners Rob Challen and Becky Playle; my grandchildren Benjamin and Otis Palmer Challen and Lauren Palmer; my siblings Kevin, Glynis, Michael, Any and Marianne Tingay. They have all been kind and supportive and put up with my absenteeism. I had told them I was retired and ready to play and then did this.

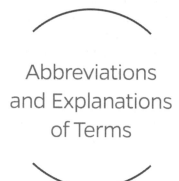

Abbreviations and Explanations of Terms

Abbreviations (organisations)

Codex Codex Alimentarius Commission
ENN Emergencies Nutrition Network
EU European Union
FAO Food and Agriculture Organisation of the United Nations
FDA Food and Drug Administration of the United States
IBFAN International Baby Food Action Network
ICDC International Code Documentation Centre
ICIFI International Council of Infant Food Industries
ILO International Labour Organisation
UN United Nations
UNICEF United Nations Children's Fund
UNHCR United Nations High Commission for Refugees
WABA World Alliance for Breastfeeding Action
WHA World Health Assembly
WHO World Health Organisation

Abbreviations (general)

BFHI Baby Friendly Hospital Initiative (in UK called BFI)

BMS Breastmilk substitute

The Code The International Code of Marketing of Breastmilk Substitutes

CRC Convention on the Rights of the Child

FOM Follow-on milk

GDP Gross Domestic Product

GI Gastrointestinal infection

GSIYCF Global Strategy for Infant and Young Child Feeding

HIV/AIDS Human immunodeficiency virus/acquired immunodeficiency syndrome

LAM Lactational Amenorrhoea Method

SCM Sweetened Condensed Milk

SDGs UN Sustainable Development Goals

PIF Powdered infant formula

RI Respiratory Infection

UNSNA United Nations System of National Accounts

General terms

Artificial feeding Any feeding method that substitutes breastfeeding. This was the standard medical term used in many text books up until the late 20th century.

Artificial milk Any milk-based product, whether commercial or home made, that is used to feed a baby or young child.

Baby A newborn or small child. The age range of the term baby varies widely according to different cultures and family custom.

Baby milk A breastmilk substitute commonly based on modified cows' milk.

Big business The large transnational commercial companies with considerable power and influence; also called multinational companies. I also use the terms corporation, industry (as in 'infant feeding industry') and manufacturers.

Breastmilk substitute Any food marketed or otherwise represented as a partial or total replacement for breastmilk, whether or not suitable for that purpose.

Company A commercial business enterprise

Infant A baby aged 0 to 12 months

Infant milk Another term for baby milk

Infant formula A term for artificial milk devised in the USA in the early 20th century as a promotional description of breastmilk substitutes. Now used in official international documents in English.

Microbe/microorganism An organism too small to be seen with the naked eye. They include bacteria and viruses.

Optimal breastfeeding Breastfeeding exclusively for the first six months of life followed by continued breastfeeding, together with nutritious family foods for two years and beyond.

Pathogen A microbe/microorganism that produces a disease.

Personalised medicine Treatment tailored to the individual patient.

Poor regions Parts of the world where large numbers of people live in poverty with inadequate access to safe water, sanitaiton and healthcare.

Rich regions Parts of the world where large numbers of people have access to safe water, sanitation and healthcare. I am aware that there are people living in so-called 'developed societies' in conditions of poverty and that in the poorest nations some citizens live in luxury, but these general terms are necessary.

Wet nursing When a woman who is not the child's mother breastfeeds a baby. This may be a commercial arrangement or done out of altruism, such as when grandmothers breastfeed orphaned grandchildren.

Young child A child aged 12 months to five years.

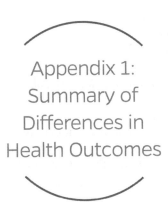

Appendix 1: Summary of Differences in Health Outcomes

List of differences in health outcomes associated with method of infant feeding (adjusted for social and economic variables). All studies were conducted in an industrialised setting.

Artificially-fed babies are at greater risk of:
· Gastro-intestinal infection
· Respiratory infections
· Necrotising enterocolitis and late onset sepsis in preterm babies
· Urinary tract infections
· Ear infections
· Allergic disease (eczema, asthma and wheezing)
· Type 1 and type 2 diabetes
· Obesity
· Childhood leukaemia
· SIDS

Breastfed babies may have better:
· Neurological development
· Cholesterol levels
· Blood pressure

Women who breastfed are at lower risk of:
· Breast cancer
· Ovarian cancer
· Hip fractures and reduced bone density

Other potential protective effects of breastfeeding (more research needed):

For the infant:
· Multiple sclerosis
· Acute appendicitis
· Tonsillectomy
· Improved parenting
· Reduced child neglect/abuse

For the mother:
· Rheumatoid arthritis
· Maternal type 2 diabetes
· Postnatal depression

Source: UNICEF UK Babyfriendly Initiative www.unicef.org.
 uk/babyfriendly

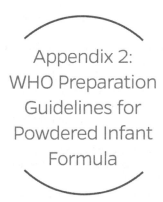

Appendix 2: WHO Preparation Guidelines for Powdered Infant Formula

Summary of the WHO guidance for preparing individual feeds in the home environment for immediate consumption.

1. Throughly clean and sterilise all feeding and preparation equipment

a) Wash hands thoroughly with soap and water before cleaning and sterilising all feeding and preparation equipment.

b) Wash feeding and preparation equipment (e.g. cups, bottles, teats and spoons) thoroughly in hot soapy water to ensure that all remaining feed is removed; rinse thoroughly in safe water.

c) After washing feeding and preparation equipment, sterilise by boiling in a large pan or using a commercial home steriliser (follow manufacturer's instructions).

d) Wash hands thoroughly with soap and water before removing feeding equipment from steriliser or pan; the use of sterilised kitchen tongs is recommended.

e) To prevent recontamination, only remove feeding and preparation equipment just before use; if not used immediately, cover and store in a clean place (fully assemble feeding bottles to prevent recontamination).

2. Freshly prepare an individual powdered infant formula feed

a) Clean and disinfect a surface on which to prepare the feed.
b) Wash hands thoroughly with soap and water and dry using a cloth or single-use napkin.
c) Boil a sufficient amount of safe water; bottled water must be boiled before use, and microwaves should never be used for preparation due to the risk of scalding.
d) Allow water to cool to no less than 70°C and pour the appropriate amount of water into a cleaned and sterilised feeding cup or bottle; water should not be left for more than 30mins after boiling.
e) To the water, add the exact amount of formula as instructed on the label; adding more or less powder than instructed could make infants ill.
f) If using bottles: assemble the cleaned and sterilised parts of the bottle according to the manufacturer's instructions; shake or swirl gently until the contents are mixed thoroughly.
g) If using feeding cups: mix thoroughly by stirring with a cleaned and sterilised spoon.

3) Quickly cool individual powdered infant formula feed to feeding temperature immediately after preparation

a) Immediately after preparation, hold bottle or feeding cup under running tap water or place in a container of cold or iced water; ensure the level of the cooling water is below the top of the cup or lid of the bottle.
b) Dry the outside of the feeding cup or bottle with a clean or disposable cloth.
c) Check the feeding temperature before feeding; this is essential to avoid the risk of scalding, and if necessary continue cooling as outlined above.
d) Discard any feed that has not been consumed within two hours.

Source: www.who.int/foodsafety/publications/powdered-infant-formula/en

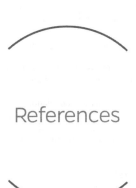

References

Preface
1. Muller M. *The Baby Killer*. London: War on Want 1974.
2. Palmer G. *The Politics of Breastfeeding: when breasts are bad for business.* (3rd edition). Pinter & Martin, 2009.

Chapter 1: What's this all about?
3. Macaskill W. *Doing Good Better: How Effective Altruism Can Help You Make A Difference.* Guardian Books, 2015.
4. Victora C.G. *et al* (2016). Breastfeeding in the 21st century: epidemiology, mechanisms, and lifelong effect. *The Lancet*, volume 387, issue 10017: 475–90.
5. Edmond K.M. *et al* (2006). Delayed breastfeeding initiation increases risk of neonatal mortality. *Paediatrics*, volume 117, issue 3: 380-6.
6. Newcomb P. *et al* (1994). Lactation and a reduced risk of postmenopausal breast cancer. *The New England Journal of Medicine*, issue 330: 81–87. As cited in Mason F., Rawe K., and Wright S. (2013). *Superfood for Babies: How overcoming barriers to breastfeeding will save children's lives.* London: The Save the Children Fund.
7. Kent G. (2015). Global infant formula: monitoring and regulating the impacts to protect human health. *International Breastfeeding Journal*, 10:6.
8. Rollins N.C. *et al* (2016). Why invest, and what it will take to improve breastfeeding practices? *The Lancet*, volume 387, issue 10017: 491-504.

Chapter 2: A good system undermined

1. Prentice A.M. *et al* (1980). Dietary supplementation of Gambian nursing mothers and lactational performance. *The Lancet*, volume 2, issue 8200: 886-8.

2. De Waal A. *Famine that kills*. Oxford Clarendon Press, 1989 and (updated) Oxford University Press, 2004.

3. Cadogan W. *An essay upon nursing and the management of children, from birth to three years of age*. London: John Knapton 1748 (first ed).

Chapter 3: Breastfeeding, fertility and population

1. Dr. Collins. *Practical Rules for the Management and Medical Treatment of Negro Slaves in the Sugar Colonies*. J Barfield, 1803.

2. Based on World Alliance of Breastfeeding Action (WABA): www.waba. org.my/resources/lam/

Chapter 4: A perfect storm

1. Edmond K.M. *et al* (2006). Delayed breastfeeding initiation increases risk of neonatal mortality. *Paediatrics*, volume 117, issue 3: 380-6.

2. Drucker P. (business and management theoretician). *Management*. New York: Harper & Row, 1974.

3. Coutts F.J.M. Inquiry into condensed milks with special reference to their use as infants' foods. *Local Government Board Reports: Food Report No.15*. London: HMSO, 1911. Also Coutts FJM. On the use of proprietary foods for infant feeding and analysis and composition of some proprietary foods for infant feeding. *Food Report No.20* London: HMSO, 1914.

4. Williams C. *Milk and Murder*. Address to the Singapore Rotary Club 1939. Allain A. (ed) Penang: IOCU, PO Box 1045, 10830 Penang, Malaysia

5. Jelliffe D.B. and Jelliffe E.F.P., *Human Milk in the Modern World*, Oxford: Oxford University Press, 1978

6. Apple R. *Mothers and medicine: a history of infant feeding from 1850–1950*. Madison: University of Wisconsin Press, 1887: p21. Also: Rotch TM. A discussion on the modification of milk in the feeding of infants. *BMJ*, 6 September 1902: 653. I am indebted to Rima Apple for her groundbreaking research and have drawn substantially on her work.

Chapter 5: A changing world

1. Chetley A. *The Baby Killer Scandal: A War on Want investigation into the promotion and sale of powdered baby milks in the Third World*. London: War on Want, 1979.

2. Willat N. How Nestlé adapts products to its markets. *Business Abroad,* June 1970: p31–3.

3. Williams C. Interview in the *Lansing Star*, 18 October 1978.

Chapter 6: Protest, action and politics

1. Jelliffe D.B. (1971). Commerciogenic malnutrition? *Food Technology*,

25: 55-56. Also: Wennen van der May CAM (1960). The decline of breastfeeding in Nigeria. *Tropical and Geographical Medicine*, 21: 93

2. Muller M. *The Baby Killer*. London: War on Want 1974

Chapter 7: Advertising is not information
1. CAC, 28th Session. Proposals of Working Group for Sectors on Food Additives, 2 Sept 2006, www.codexalimentarius.net
2. Crawley H. and Westland S., *Infant Milks in the UK: A Practical Guide for Health Professionals*. First Steps Nutrition Trust, June 2015 and Crawley H. and Westland S., *Scientific and factual? A review of breastmilk substitute advertising to healthcare professionals*. First Steps Nutrition Trust, 2016
3. Kent G. (2015). Global infant formula: monitoring and regulating the impacts to protect human health. *International Breastfeeding Journal*, 10:6

Chapter 8: A reality check
1. Walters D. *et al* (2016). The Cost of Not Breastfeeding in Southeast Asia. *Health, Policy and Planning*, 1-10. Plus personal communication Roger Mathisen.
2. 'A Tightening Grip'. *The Economist*. March 14, 2015.
3. Walters D. *et al* (2016). The Cost of Not Breastfeeding in Southeast Asia. *Health, Policy and Planning*, 1-10. Plus personal communication Roger Mathisen.
4. Euromonitor: Global Packaged Food: Market Opportunities for Baby Food to 2013. Sept 2008.
5. WHO and UNICEF Joint Monitoring Programme 2015. Progress on Drinking Water and Sanitation. 2015 Update and MDG Assessment.

Chapter 9: Dying for the code
1. See Brazilian Government's website: www.brasil.gov.br/cidadania-e-justica/2015/09/brasil-esta-acima-da-media-mundial-na-reducao-da-mortalidade-infantil-diz-onu.
2. Clavano N.R. *The results of a change in hospital practices – a paeditrican's campaign for breastfeeding in the Philippines. A Case Study.* Assignment Children 55/56, UNICEF, 1981. NB: Dr Clavano was a witness at the 1978 US Senate Hearing.
3. See www.who.int/nutrition/publications/infantfeeding/9241562218/en/
4. *Formula for Disaster* (film) UNICEF 2007. May be viewed online at www.babymilkaction.org.

Chapter 10: Value for money
1. Laslett P. *The World we have lost - further explored*. London: Methuen, 1983.
2. Campbell C.E. (1984). Nestlé and breast vs bottle-feeding: mainstream and Marxist perspectives. *International Journal of Health Services*, volume 14,

issue 4: 547-66.
3. Estimate by Bank of England economics cited in George S, *The Lugano Report II*, Transnational Institute, Amsterdam 2013
4. NY Attorney General Office Report, cited in *NY Times* and *The Lugano Report II* cited above.
5. Lanchester J. When Bitcoin Grows Up. *London Review of Books*, 21 April 2016.
6. *Global Food: Waste Not, Want Not.* Report by Fox T, Head of Energy and Environment, IMECHE. UK, January 2013.
7. Aguayo V.M. and Ross J. (2002). The monetary value of human milk in Francophone West Africa: a profile for nutrition policy communication. *Food and Nutrition Bulletin*, volume 23, issue 2: 153-161.
8. Waring M. *If women counted: a new feminist economics.* Macmillan, 1988. Also an expanded and updated version of this book. *Counting for nothing: What men value and what women are worth.* University of Toronto Press, 1999.
9. Smith J.P. and Ingham L.H. (2005). Mothers' milk and Measures of Economic Output. *Feminist Economics*, volume 11, issue 1: 41-62.
10. See *The Lancet Series on Breastfeeding*: Rollins N.C. et al (2016). Why invest, and what it will take to improve breastfeeding practices? *The Lancet*, volume 387, issue 10017: 491-504. Also: Victora C.G. et al (2016). Breastfeeding in the 21st century: epidemiology, mechanisms, and lifelong effect. *The Lancet*, volume 387, issue 10017: 475–90.

Chapter 11: Women's work

1. National Domestic Workers Alliance cited in Aviv R., The Cost of Caring. *New Yorker*, April 11, 2016.
2. North A., The Dark Underworld of Bangladesh's Clothing Industry, BBC Online, 26 April 2013.
3. The UN Research Institute for Social Development (UNRISD). *States of disarray: the social effects of globalisation.* UNRISD, 1995 [p70 350,000 illegal nannies in the USA.] Also: Parreñas R. *The Global Servants: (Im)Migrant Filipina Domnestic Workers in Rome and Los Angeles* PhD dissertation, Dpt. Of Ethnic Studies, UCal, Berkeley, 1999, in Hochschild AR, Love and Gold in Ehrenreich B. and Hochschild A.R., *Global Women, Nannies, Maids and Sex workers in the New Economy.* Granta Books, 2003.
4. Professor Maria Ibarra of San Diego State University cited in Aviv R, The Cost of Caring. *The New Yorker*, April 11, 2016.
5. Winikof B. and Laukaren V.H. (1989). Breastfeeding and Bottlefeeding Controversies in the Developing World: Evidence from a Study in Four Countries. *Social Science and Medicine*, 29: 859-868.

Chapter 12: The big issues

1. Sen A. *Poverty and Famines: An Essay on Entitlement and Deprivation.* Oxford New York: Clarendon Press Oxford University Press, 1982.

2. Kent G. (2015). Global infant formula: monitoring and regulating the impacts to protect human health. *International Breastfeeding Journal*, 10:6.

3. Figures and facts from Valerie Gatchell and Caroline Wilkinsons of UNHCR, and Marie McGrath of ENN, 2016.

4. Bailey L. *et al* (2014). Association of Antibiotics in Infancy with Early Childhood Obesity. JAMA Paediatrics, volume 168, issue 11: 1063-1069. Also see Saari A *et al* (2015). Antibiotic Exposure in Infancy and Risk of Being Overweight in the First 24 Months of Life. *Paediatrics*, volume 135, issue 4: 617-626.

5. Ashley B. *et al*. Global prevalence of antibiotic resistance in paediatric urinary tract infections caused by E coli and association with routine use of antibiotics in primary care: systematic review and meta-analysis. *BMJ*, March 2016, 352.

6. Titmuss R.M (1997) *The Gift Relationship*. LSE Books.

7. UK Chief Medical Officer, Dame Sally Davies: Annual Report 2016.

8. Report on Carbon Footprint due to Milk Formula. A study from selected countries of the Asia-Pacific Region. BPNI/IBFAN Asia. *IBFAN*, 2015.

9. waronwant.org/ttip

10. Wilkinson R. and Pickett K., *The Spirit Level: Why more equal societies almost always do better*. Penguin Books, 2009.

11. Article 57 Convention on the Rights of the Child. See www.unicef.org/crc

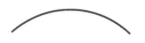

Useful Contacts

Emergencies Nutrition Network (ENN) www.ennonline.net

Food First Information and Action Network (FIAN)
www.fian.org

International Baby Food Action Network (IBFAN)
www.ibfan.org

International Labour Organisation (ILO) www.ilo.org

International Lactation Consultants' Association (ILCA)
www.ilca.org

La Leche League International (LLLI) www.llli.org

People's Health Movement www.phmovement.org

UNICEF www.unicef.org

World Alliance for Breastfeeding Action (WABA)
www.waba.org.my

WHO www.who.org

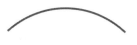

Index

Index